1993

THE REFORM OF HEALTH CARE

*A Comparative Analysis
of Seven OECD Countries*

ORGANISATION FOR ECONOMIC CO-OPERATION AND DEVELOPMENT

ORGANISATION FOR ECONOMIC CO-OPERATION AND DEVELOPMENT

Pursuant to Article 1 of the Convention signed in Paris on 14th December 1960, and which came into force on 30th September 1961, the Organisation for Economic Co-operation and Development (OECD) shall promote policies designed:

— to achieve the highest sustainable economic growth and employment and a rising standard of living in Member countries, while maintaining financial stability, and thus to contribute to the development of the world economy;

— to contribute to sound economic expansion in Member as well as non-member countries in the process of economic development; and

— to contribute to the expansion of world trade on a multilateral, non-discriminatory basis in accordance with international obligations.

The original Member countries of the OECD are Austria, Belgium, Canada, Denmark, France, Germany, Greece, Iceland, Ireland, Italy, Luxembourg, the Netherlands, Norway, Portugal, Spain, Sweden, Switzerland, Turkey, the United Kingdom and the United States. The following countries became Members subsequently through accession at the dates indicated hereafter: Japan (28th April 1964), Finland (28th January 1969), Australia (7th June 1971) and New Zealand (29th May 1973). The Commission of the European Communities takes part in the work of the OECD (Article 13 of the OECD Convention).

Publié en français sous le titre :

LA RÉFORME DES SYSTÈMES DE SANTÉ
ANALYSE COMPARÉE
DE SEPT PAYS DE L'OCDE

FOREWORD

To achieve government objectives, reforms are almost always necessary. Policy designers do not – indeed, cannot – foresee all behavioural responses of complex systems. The external environment evolves in unpredictable ways.

In health systems, as elsewhere, reforms are something of a permanent feature. The real question is: why such a book?

In terms of ambition and scope, policy reforms conceived or initiated during the past five years exceed the reforms of the preceding two or three decades. The earlier reforms had already been important, as the road towards universal access and responsible financing is anything but smooth. The delivery systems had to adjust to rapidly expanding technology and to equally rapid ''medical demography''. The private/public mix faced strains at times but, by and large, the OECD health systems coped, with reasonable success.

One thing that *is* predictable is change: new challenges bring with them new strains on the systems. Rejuvenation and incentives are again needed if we are to surpass the efficiency standards attained.

In health, as in other policy domains, the OECD has a permanent policy monitoring function. Under the auspices of its Working Party on Social Policy, an analysis of the sizeable reforms is under way. This study reports on the first phase of that work; it covers seven European countries: Belgium, France, Germany, Ireland, the Netherlands, Spain, the United Kingdom. The second phase looks at other countries.

The analysis reveals that Member states all face much the same problems regarding management of their health systems – which was partly to be expected. More revealing, however, is the surprisingly high degree of convergence in the goals pursued, the similarity of approaches taken and that these similarities occur without losing sight of cultural diversity or national institutions. It should be noted that this convergence is not the result of any prior international concertation.

Within the countries examined, much experimentation was to be found, albeit around common themes and under the constraint of fiscal frugality.

This report was prepared in 1989-1990 by Jeremy Hurst, Senior Economic Adviser in the British Department of Health. Jeremy Hurst is indebted to many experts, government officials, academics, and others, who supplied much background material and significant comments on early drafts. The OECD Secretariat updated the institutional development through mid-1992, before publication.

This report is published on the responsibility of the OECD Secretary-General.

T. J. Alexander
Director for Education, Employment,
Labour and Social Affairs OECD

ALSO AVAILABLE

The Future of Social Protection. Series OECD Social Policy Studies. No. 6 (1988)
(81 88 03 1) ISBN 92-64-13152-3   FF70   £8.50   US$15.50   DM31

Health Care Systems in Transition: The Search for Efficiency. Series OECD Social Policy Studies. No. 7 (1990)
(81 89 05 1) ISBN 92-64-13310-0   FF140   £17.00 US$30.00   DM55

Living Conditions in OECD Countries: Compendium of Social Indicators. Series OECD Social Policy Studies. No. 3 (1986)
(81 85 04 1) ISBN 92-64-12734-8   FF65   £6.50   US$13.00   DM29

Contents

SUMMARY

OECD Member countries continue to face persistent difficulties in the financing and delivery of their health services. The problems, which vary between countries, include:

- Remaining gaps in access to services, and in income protection when medical care is required;
- Unacceptably rapid increases in health expenditure and;
- Concerns about inefficiency and poor performance.

Partly, these difficulties are the result of circumstances – for example, demographic and technological change – which are mainly or partly outside the control of governments. To some extent however, they arise from remediable flaws in the way in which the financing, payment and regulation systems for health care are designed.

This report covers a comparative investigation of health care reforms introduced during the 1980s in seven OECD countries: Belgium, France, Germany, Ireland, the Netherlands, Spain, and the United Kingdom. The focus is on reforms because it is at times of reform that policy-makers think carefully about their objectives for health care, about the problems which they are experiencing, as well as the best solutions.

At first sight, the prospects for making comparisons across these seven OECD countries appear to be slight. There seems to be great diversity in their health care financing and delivery institutions. However, closer investigation suggests that all seven health care systems are made up from different mixtures of a handful of sub-systems, found repeatedly across these and other OECD countries. Moreover, most of the seven health care systems are dominated by just one or two of these sub-systems.

Apart from direct, out-of-pocket payments, six major sub-systems which involve third-party payment can be identified. These comprise combinations of two major sources of finance for third-party payment:

 i) Voluntary (or private) premiums; and
 ii) Compulsory (or public) contributions or taxes;

as well as three methods by which the third parties can arrange for benefits to be provided:

 a) Reimbursement of patients for medical bills (indemnity insurance) with no connection between insurers and providers;
 b) Direct contracts with providers, who are often independent, usually with work-related payment systems;
 c) Ownership and management of providers in an integrated model, generally lacking work-related payment systems.

During the 1980s, the health care systems of all seven countries were dominated by one or more of the three sub-systems which involve compulsory finance.

Belgium relied on a blend of the public reimbursement (of patients) model and the public contract model.

France relied on a blend of the public reimbursement, contract and integrated models.

The Federal Republic of Germany and *the Netherlands* relied mainly on the public contract model.

Ireland and *the United Kingdom* relied on a mixture of the public contract and integrated models.

The Länder of the Eastern part of Germany and *Spain* relied mainly on the public integrated model.

Voluntary health insurance accounted for no more than 15 % of health expenditure in any of the countries.

The difficulties experienced by each country tended to depend on which sub-systems of finance and delivery dominated:

- Systems which still relied on vestiges of the public reimbursement model tended to have most difficulties with cost containment;
- Countries which relied on the public contract model often suffered from lack of competition and excessive regulation;

- Countries which relied on the public integrated model tended to suffer from managerial inadequacies and failures of responsiveness to consumers.

All seven countries initiated moderate or major reforms to their health care systems during the 1980s.

Several countries, particularly Spain, the Netherlands and Ireland, took further steps to extend eligibility for public medical care, bringing the last remaining groups of their populations into the public system of coverage for basic medical care. Despite widespread calls for privatisation of finance, none of the other countries took significant steps to reduce their commitment to public coverage.

Several countries took important initiatives in the field of cost containment. In most cases, governments resorted to some extent to increased cost-sharing. However, most of the reforms aimed at containing costs were concentrated on the supply side. This involved the determined application of prospective, global budgets, especially for hospital expenditure in Belgium, France, Germany and the Netherlands. Compared with the 1970s, all seven countries greatly reduced the rate of growth of their health expenditures during the 1980s. Those countries which still relied, to some extent, on the public reimbursement model were rather less successful in this respect than those which relied on the public contract and integrated models.

Perhaps the most important reforms of the 1980s involved the introduction of improved incentives and regulations for providers and insurers, with the aim of raising the productivity of rationed resources. It is possible to distinguish three separate sets of developments.

- There was some convergence on the public contract model. Belgium and France introduced tighter contracts into their reimbursement models, and the United Kingdom and the Länder of East Germany abandoned their integrated models in favour of contract models.
- Some countries embarked on reforms to the contract model itself, by placing a fresh emphasis on: consumer choice; active, informed purchasing rather than passive funding by third parties; and on managed competition between providers. This was clearest in Germany, but elements of such changes were also seen in Belgium and in the Netherlands. The new contracting models are characterised by mixed payment systems, which combine budgetary caps with work-related payment of providers. The expectation is that, by enabling governments to stand back somewhat, more self-regulation will be possible.
- Finally, two countries – the Netherlands and the United Kingdom – embarked on experiments which involve the introduction of competition between third parties within their public systems. The two experiments are rather different. In the Netherlands it is envisaged that consumers will be able to choose between sickness funds and private insurers, with a central health care fund taking in income-related premiums and paying out risk-related premiums to the competing insurers. This amounts to a sophisti- cated health voucher scheme. The experiment in the United Kingdom involves giving part of the hospital budget to some, large (competing) general practices. This will enable general practitioners to purchase certain hospital services on behalf of their patients.

This last set of reforms is particularly controversial. The reforms are also only gradually introduced in the Netherlands and are recent in the United Kingdom. For this reason, it is not yet possible to gauge their full results. However, there are already signs that general practitioner "fundholders" in the United Kingdom are using their new purchasing power to negotiate a higher quality of hospital services for their patients.

GLOSSARY

This glossary provides definitions of some of the key terms used in this report.

Accreditation: the process by which an agency or organisation evaluates and recognises an institution as meeting certain professional standards.

Agency model: the relationship between patient and doctor in which the doctor supplies technical expertise and subordinates his or her own interests to the interests of the patient when diagnosing, prescribing and treating.

Basic health care: a minimum set, or core, of health services.

Benefits: in health insurance, either a payment in cash paid in settlement of a claim under the terms of an indemnity policy or the provision of a service in kind following a medical contingency covered by a scheme.

Bilateral monopoly: a market in which a single buyer faces a single seller.

Capitation payment: a fixed payment to a provider for each listed or enrolled person served per period of time. Payments will vary according to the number of patients enrolled but not with the number of services rendered per patient.

Co-insurance: cost-sharing in the form of a set proportion of the cost of a service. In France and Belgium, *"ticket modérateur"*.

Command and control: either, government regulation of a health care market by detailed central planning and fixing of prices, quantities and capacity; or, government regulation of a public integrated health care system via line management. The aim is generally to plan and manage the allocation of resources and to pursue efficiency objectives without relying on markets or competition.

Competition: rivalry between two or more sellers for revenue, market share or other advantage.

Compulsory health insurance: health insurance under an obligatory public scheme. Payment for such insurance amounts to a tax. The obligation may be placed on an employer to pay contributions on behalf of his or her employees. Contributions are usually income-related. Compulsory insurance is usually administered by public bodies, but it can be administered by private insurance carriers, as is the case with the scheme for civil servants in the Netherlands.

Contract model: the term used in this study for compulsory or voluntary health insurance which involves direct payments, under contract, from the insurers or third parties to the providers for services rendered to insured persons (see Charts 2.4 and 2.5, Chapter 2). This means that benefits are supplied in kind to patients, often free of charge. In this model the providers are often independent and the contractual payments to them are often by capitation or by fee for service. In the United States, two voluntary forms of this model are known respectively as the group practice model and the individual practice model of the health maintenance organisation.

Contribution: tax payment levied for compulsory health insurance, often as part of a social security scheme. May be split between employer and employee. Often set at a fixed proportion of income between a floor and ceiling level of income.

Co-payment: cost-sharing in the form of a fixed amount to be paid for a service.

Cost-sharing: a provision of health insurance or third-party payment that requires the individual who is covered to pay part of the cost of medical care received. This is distinct from the payment of a health insurance premium, contribution or tax which is paid whether medical care is received or not. Cost-sharing may be in the form of deductibles, co-insurance or co-payments.

Countervailing power: for example, the use of concentrated buying power to counteract monopoly power.

Deductible: cost-sharing in the form of a fixed amount which must be paid for a service before any payment of benefits can take place.

Externalities: (spillover effects) costs or benefits which arise from production or consumption; which fall on individuals and groups not directly involved in the production or consumption concerned; and which are not compensated for by exchange. For example, immunisation of an individual against an infectious disease can block the transmission of the disease to other individuals who are not directly involved and who pay nothing for the protection which they receive. This creates an external benefit.

Extra billing: additional charges levied by providers on patients over and above: agreed indemnity payments, or contracted fees, and any cost-sharing pre-arranged by the third parties. Extra billing is a likely by-product of the reimbursement model and physician monopoly power (or an inelastic supply) because patients' ability to pay is augmented by insurance.

Fee for service: payments to a provider for each act or service rendered.

Global budget: (used as a shorthand for "prospective global budget") an aggregate cash sum, fixed in advance, intended to cover the total cost of a service, usually for one year ahead.

Health outcome: changes in health status (mortality and morbidity) which result from the provision of health (or other) services.

Indemnity insurance: see "reimbursement model".

Integrated model: the term used in this report for compulsory or voluntary health insurance or third-party funding in which both the insurance and provision of health care is supplied by the same organisation in a vertically integrated system (see Charts 2.6 and 2.7, Chapter 2). In this model, doctors are typically paid by salary and hospitals are typically funded by global budgets. As in the contract model, benefits are supplied to patients in kind, often free of charge. In the United States, the voluntary form of this model is better known as the staff model of the health maintenance organisation. The public version of this model involves government financing and provision of health care and is often funded mainly out of general taxation.

Managed competition: government regulation of a health care market which uses competition as the means to achieve efficiency objectives within a framework of government intervention designed to achieve other policy objectives, such as equity.

Monopolist: a single seller.

Monopsonist: a single buyer.

Moral hazard: the tendency for insurance cover to: encourage risk-taking behaviour by the insured individual and to raise his or her demand for health (or repair) services by lowering the net price of such services. These hazards increase the risk to the insurer and, if not checked, are likely to lead to higher claims and higher insurance premiums.

Mutuelles and Mutualités: private, non-profit health insurers, or friendly societies, in France and Belgium, respectively.

Oligopoly: few sellers.

Open enrolment: a period during which an insurer may be required to take any new member or subscriber irrespective of their risk.

Out-of-pocket payments: payments borne directly by a patient without the benefit of insurance. They include cost-sharing.

Premium: payment for voluntary insurance. Premiums may be risk-related (tailored to the actuarial risk or claims experience for each individual) or they may be flat rate or community-rated (averaged across a group of individuals).

Private health insurance: see "voluntary health insurance".

Progressive taxation: a tax which takes an increasing proportion of income as income rises.

Public health insurance: see "compulsory health insurance".

Regressive taxation: a tax which takes a declining proportion of income as income rises.

Regulation: intervention by government, by means of rules, in health care markets or systems. There are two main types of regulation: pro-competitive or pro-market regulation (generally with encouragement of choice among consumers, and of autonomy and competition among insurers and/or providers); and command-and-control regulation (often with discouragement of choice among consumers, and of autonomy and competition among insurers and/or providers).

Reimbursement model: the term used in this study for compulsory or voluntary health insurance involving cash reimbursement of patients for all or part of the cost of medical care received. Otherwise known as "indemnity insurance" (see Charts 2.2 and 2.3, Chapter 2). In the pure form of this model there is no connection between the third parties and the providers.

Risk selection: the process by which insurers (or providers) who are paid a flat, or non-risk-related, premium (or capitation payment) seek to encourage custom from individuals with below-average risk and discourage or refuse custom from individuals with above-average risk.

Salary payment: remuneration which is fixed per period of time and does not vary either with the number of individuals served or with the number of services rendered.

Social assistance model: model under which the availability of health benefits under a public, third-party scheme depends on an income or a wealth test.

Social health insurance: a term mainly used to denote compulsory, or public, health insurance, usually part of a social security system, which is funded from specific (mainly payroll) contributions and is managed by autonomous or quasi autonomous sickness funds, friendly societies or private insurers.

Solidarity: a term used mainly in European countries which denotes compulsory risk pooling in a public health insurance scheme, with payment for health care based on ability to pay and the offer of health care based on medical need.

Supplier-induced demand: the supposed ability of doctors to boost the demand for their services or for the services of colleagues.

Third-party payer: any organisation, public or private, that pays or insures health care expenses for beneficiaries at the time at which they are patients. The first party is the patient and the second party is the provider. Third parties may be: private insurers; quasi public bodies, such as sickness funds; and government bodies themselves.

Ticket modérateur: see "co-insurance".

Voluntary health insurance: health insurance which is taken up and paid for at the discretion of individuals, or employers on behalf of individuals. Voluntary insurance can be offered by a public or quasi public body, as is the case in Ireland.

Work-related payment: see "fee for service" and "capitation payment".

Yardstick competition: comparisons of the price and quality of specific goods and services offered by monopolists or oligopolists in local markets, with the price and quality of similar goods and services in distant markets. Although there may be no direct competition between local and distant markets, such comparisons may reveal the potential scope for competition and may be useful to a purchaser in bargaining, or to a regulatory authority in promoting competitive behaviour.

Reference

U.S. House of Representatives (1976), *A Discursive Dictionary of Health Care,* U.S. Government Printing Office, Washington, 1976.

Chapter 1

INTRODUCTION AND MAIN ISSUES

INTRODUCTION

OECD Member countries continue to face persistent difficulties with the financing, delivery and performance of their health care systems, despite the successful implementation of new policies since the mid-1970s. This report considers the ways in which these problems are being tackled in seven OECD countries. It is addressed to governments in OECD countries in general because of the responsibilities which they all carry for the financing, regulation and provision of health services.

The report approaches these issues through a comparison of recent and prospective reforms to the health care systems in the selected OECD countries. Usually, much may be learned when countries reform their health care systems. This is a time when policy-makers think carefully about objectives, about existing health care institutions, about the causes of the problems which face them and about the available solutions. Despite the well documented differences which exist between countries in medical culture (Payer, 1989), in health care institutions (Raffel, 1984), and in medical practice itself (McPherson, 1989), international comparisons of subsequent reforms can shed light on common problems and common solutions. OECD countries share similar health policy objectives; the apparent diversity in their health care financing and organisation arrangements disguises the fact that each system is made up from a fairly short list of sub-systems, a few of which tend to dominate. These points will be developed more fully in this chapter and in the chapter which follows.

The countries which were selected for this study are all in Western Europe. They were chosen for a mixture of reasons including: the importance of the reforms they had made in the 1980s or were contemplating in the 1990s; the extent to which they represent the different types of health care system found among OECD countries; the willingness of their administrations to participate in the study; and the economy of conducting the investigations in one continent. In addition, the study draws on experience from North America. The countries fall into three main groups which represent most of the main health care systems found in OECD Member countries:

The Netherlands	financed by a mixture of social and private insurance, with mainly private providers;
Belgium, France and Germany	financed mainly by social insurance, with mixed private and public providers;
Ireland, Spain and the United Kingdom	financed mainly by general taxation, with mainly public providers.

An important distinction in health policy has to be made between the production of health services and the production of health itself. The health of the population depends not only on health care, but also on many other factors which include standards of living, housing, life-styles, diet and environmental circumstances. This study confines itself to the production of health services, and to the effect which those services have on the health of the population, other things being equal. In other words, the study concentrates on the financing, organisation and results of preventive medical care, primary medical care and hospital care – all forms of care which involve doctors, nurses and other medical and paramedical professionals. The study does not deal with health promotion in the wider sense or with dental care. Neither does it consider in any great depth the arrangements for long-term care, particularly those at the boundaries between health services and social services.

The purpose of this chapter is:

- To set out some of the main objectives of health care policy;
- To discuss the strengths and weaknesses of free markets and government institutions for health care; and
- To introduce some current problems with the financing and delivery of health care in the countries included in this study.

Chapter 2 goes on to discuss some main sub-systems of financing and delivery of care. The seven health care systems themselves and their recent reforms are described in some detail in Chapters 3 to 9. Chapter 10 contains statistical comparisons on the growth and performance of the health care systems in the seven countries. Chapter 11 compares and appraises the reforms, and Chapter 12 is devoted to policy conclusions.

COMMON OBJECTIVES OF HEALTH CARE POLICY

The seven countries appear to share similar objectives in their health care policies. Stated briefly, and drawing on Barr (1990), these include:

Adequacy and equity in access to care: there should be some minimum of health care available to all citizens and treatment should be in accordance with need, at least in the publicly financed sector.

Income protection: patients should be protected from payments for health care which threaten income sufficiency and the payment for protection should be related to individuals' ability to pay. This will involve at least three types of transfer: insurance (the need for care is unpredictable); saving (the elderly use more services than the young) and income redistribution (the sick are often the poor).

Macro-economic efficiency: health expenditure should consume an appropriate fraction of GDP.

Micro-economic efficiency: a mix of services should be chosen which maximises a combination of health outcome and consumer satisfaction for the available share of GDP expended on health services (allocative efficiency). In addition, costs should be minimised for the available share (technical and cost efficiency). The benefits should take account not only of the health of the individual patient, but also of his or her satisfaction with the method of delivering the service, and of the health and welfare of others who are likely to be affected by the patient's condition. The costs should take account not only of the costs of provision but also of the value of the time of patients and their relatives, and of the costs of administration, regulation and tax distortions. Furthermore, dynamic efficiency should be pursued: that is to say, there should be a search for technological and organisational advances which raise the productivity of given resources.

Freedom of choice for consumers: freedom of choice should be available in public sector as well as in private sector arrangements;

Appropriate autonomy for providers: doctors and other providers should be given the maximum freedom compatible with attainment of the above objectives, especially in matters of medical and organisational innovation.

The last two objectives could be treated as means rather than ends: they are included here because they have some claim to be treated as desiderata in their own right.

It goes without saying, perhaps, that these objectives involve making judgments about values which will vary between and within countries. Also, some of these objectives conflict, some overlap, and opinion will vary as to the relative priority that should be accorded to achieving any one of them.

STRENGTHS AND WEAKNESSES OF FREE MARKETS

In many sectors of OECD economies, the objectives set out above would be met by reliance on the free market, combined with general measures of income redistribution. After all, the competitive market with income redistribution is, in many areas of the economy, the most successful way which has yet been devised for combining consumer choice, producer autonomy, economic efficiency and equity. In a competitive market, the consumer is motivated to balance the benefits gained from the consumption of goods and services against the price that has to be paid for them; the profit-maximising producer has an incentive to maximise the perceived worth of the product and to minimise the cost. Competition will ensure that prices are related closely to opportunity costs – at least in the long run. The value of output will be maximised for a given distribution of income.

It may be added that, in a world with frequent technological and organisational change, allowing temporary monopolies created by innovations can help to spur dynamic, efficiency improvements. The competitive market might seem, at first glance, to be entirely appropriate for health care, too. Health care is mainly a personal service which can be provided by potentially competing professionals and private institutions. Few, important production externalities occur except in the case of infectious diseases which, with the exception of AIDS, are of dwindling importance.

However, special characteristics of the demand for and supply of health care have discouraged, and presumably always will discourage, OECD countries from relying solely on the free market combined with income redistribution for the provision of health services (Culyer, 1989).

First, the requirement for income redistribution is particularly pressing where health care is concerned. This is because opinion is widespread and firmly held that medical care of good quality should be available to all who need it without their suffering an unacceptable financial burden: there are "caring externalities". Moreover, a strong inverse relationship often exists between ill-health and the ability to pay for health care. Private charity is unlikely to provide an adequate means of meeting this demand for altruism, partly because of the "free rider" problem: each individual is tempted to leave the burden of giving to others.

Second, the need for health care is often highly unpredictable and very costly for the individual, although it is predictable and affordable for large groups. Insurance can be used to help to spread the burden of payment but private insurers will have an incentive to exclude, or raise premiums against, high-risk individuals – that is to say against those who are most sick, who will often be those with the lowest income (risk selection and premium loading). In general, those with pre-existing conditions will be refused insurance for these conditions. It is not easy to devise income redistribution mechanisms based on market principles which can cope with this. Moreover, health insurance brings a tendency towards over-consumption. Neither the patient nor the doctor has an adequate incentive to economise when a third party is paying the bill (moral hazard). Although private institutions such as health maintenance organisations have been devised to tackle moral hazard, they do not seem to be capable, in themselves, of tackling risk selection.

Third, the consumer is in a weak position in the market for health care. This is partly a result of asymmetry of knowledge. The consumer may know when he or she feels sick but is usually too ignorant to judge what can best be provided by way of remedies and to judge retrospectively the quality of care, because of the complexity of medical technology and the relative infrequency of much consumption. In addition, sickness can itself impair judgment. For these reasons, the consumer is obliged to rely heavily on the advice of the doctor and to obtain medical approval for making most major consumption decisions. In these circumstances, it is often the doctor who takes the decisions. It is not easy to maintain consumer sovereignty in these circumstances.

Whereas other markets for goods and services possess one or two of these characteristics, few, if any, possess all three.

STRENGTHS AND WEAKNESSES OF GOVERNMENT INSTITUTIONS

The difficulties with relying on the private market for health care have encouraged governments – to a greater or lesser extent – to intervene in the financing and delivery of health care. However, whereas government actions may cure or moderate the original defects to which they were addressed, they often bring unwanted side effects.

One widespread form of intervention has been the introduction of public financing of basic health care, for some or all of the population. This has been done, for example, by means of compulsory health insurance schemes financed by income-related contributions. Schemes can include low income and vulnerable groups, often with the help of tax subsidies. Such arrangements can be very successful in improving access to health care and income protection for disadvantaged groups. However, they have often succeeded at the expense of unacceptably high levels and rates of increase of public expenditure. This has been especially true when they have been developed in the shadow of private health insurance schemes.

Another common form of intervention, often introduced, in part, to tackle the side effects of the first, has been government regulation of private or mixed markets of health insurers and providers. To some extent, governments have encouraged self-regulation. For example, one early and crucial development in most countries was the professionalisation of doctors and other highly skilled health care workers. Governments granted doctors and other health professionals certain privileges of self-regulation and a collective monopoly of supply, in exchange for the adoption of ethical forms of practice and the maintenance of certain standards of qualification and practice. In addition, governments have promoted self-regulation by pro-market, or pro-competition policies. To a considerable extent, however, regulation has been of the command-and-control type, with centralised attempts to limit the rate of rise of insurance premiums, to fix the prices, quantities and quality of health services and to plan and control capacity. Such regulation seems to be capable of controlling costs, if it is applied with sufficient determination. However, it suffers from well known tendencies to become over-bureaucratic, to impose distortions and rigidities on markets and to suffer capture by the regulated industry. Where medicine is concerned, government sovereignty appears to be no more straightforward than consumer sovereignty.

Finally, governments have often chosen both to finance and to provide health care for vulnerable groups or whole populations, with salaried doctors employed in public clinics and hospitals. This can be combined with more or less autonomy on clinical matters for the doctors. These arrangements have enjoyed a mixed history in different countries. At best, they seem to be capable of supplying good quality health care according to clinical need, financed at a reasonable cost. However, they are frequently attended by waiting lists and seem to encourage a brisk and impersonal style of service. At worst, the result is over-loaded and low-quality services which are supplied by ill-motivated staff in shabby premises. It is also not unknown for publicly financed and provided health services to be corrupted by private, ''under the table'' payments from patients to professionals. While this report was being written, the former communist countries of Central and Eastern Europe were beginning to dismantle their monolithic and autocratic, state-financed and provided health services in favour of more liberal arrangements. The case of Eastern Germany is considered in Chapter 5.

CURRENT PROBLEMS WITH THE FINANCING AND DELIVERY OF HEALTH CARE

The seven countries in this study have already had much experience in trying to devise health care financing and delivery arrangements which combine the strengths of the market with the strengths of government institutions, while avoiding the weaknesses of both. The mixture of arrangements which they have chosen have enabled them to achieve some of their policy objectives for health care. Nevertheless, to judge by the scale of the reforms introduced in the 1980s, not to mention the policy debate which surrounds them, most of the governments are not, as yet, satisfied with the performance of their health care systems.

All seven countries have achieved universal, or near universal, access to basic health care of a high quality, which is largely independent of patients' ability to pay. Most are now enjoying some success in controlling costs. However, despite these achievements, all seven continue to wrestle with a range of difficulties which concern the efficiency, cost and equity of health care delivery and finance. These vary in their incidence between countries but they include:

- Continuing rapid growth of health expenditure in some and pressures for higher expenditure in all countries;
- Concern about excessive or unnecessary care and over-medicalisation of social problems in some countries;
- Concern about inadequate care and impersonal care and lack of responsiveness by providers in some countries;
- Continuing growth in queues and waiting times in some countries;
- Evidence about large and inexplicable variations in activity and unit costs between and within countries;
- Concern about lack of co-ordination among providers in most countries;
- Evidence about remaining inequities in health, in access to health care and in payment for health care in several countries.

Some of the circumstances which are believed to be causing these problems lie more or less outside the control of governments. Others appear to lie within the control of governments and to be amenable, at least potentially, to the process of reform. Others seem to occupy an intermediate position.

More or less outside the control of government are:

- Variations in the health of individuals which are the result of biological, cultural and social factors;
- The ageing of the population, which tends to raise costs because the elderly are the heaviest users of services;
- Rising expectations about standards of medical care which affect publicly funded services; and
- The continuing advance of cost-increasing medical technology.

In varying degrees, these affect all OECD countries.

The continuing paucity of information on the final product of health services – in other words, how health services affect health itself – is one area which seems to lie only partly within the competence of government. This is perhaps the main obstacle to the better management, and indeed to the reform, of health care systems. Whether this arises from difficulties with the technology for measuring health outcome, or from the way in which clinical information is monopolised by the medical profession, is open to debate. Again, lack of information about the effectiveness of health services affects all OECD countries.

Among those factors which seem to lie mainly within the competence of governments and which can be tackled by reforms are:

- Inappropriate financial incentives for providers;
- Harmful monopolistic and restrictive practices exercised by providers;
- Unsuitable organisational and management structures;
- Poorly designed regulation mechanisms; and
- Remediable gaps in information about effectiveness and costs.

The precise problems, here, vary between the countries and it is in areas such as these that governments have concentrated their reform efforts.

However, although these factors are potentially amenable to reform, governments are hampered in tackling them by their incomplete understanding of what combination of incentives and regulations best motivates providers. No entirely reliable guide exists as to the behaviour of doctors or large non-profit organisations such as hospitals. In the case of doctors, at least three plausible models of their behaviour have been advanced (Tussing, 1985):

- The "agency" model, in which the doctor supplies technical expertise and acts solely in the interests of the patient. In the case of out-of-pocket payment, this will include helping the patient to choose treatments which balance the likely benefits of care against the likely costs;
- The self-interest model, in which the doctor is motivated significantly by the desire to maximise some combination of his or her own income and leisure;
- The medical ethics model, where the doctor is motivated primarily by the desire to do as much as possible for the individual patient at hand, irrespective of the cost.

The study proceeds on the assumption that the behaviour of most physicians is driven by a mixture of these motives. Accordingly, much of the report is concerned with the search for arrangements which will reward doctors and other providers, both financially and professionally, for pursuing their traditional concern with the welfare of patients and for taking account of costs. In other words, it is concerned with encouraging behaviour which is cost-effective from the point of view of society. Fortunately, it can be shown that there is no inevitability of conflict between medical ethics and economic efficiency (Williams, 1989).

Governments are also handicapped in introducing reforms by formidable political obstacles to change and by difficulties with implementing reforms in large public systems. Even when they are convinced about the technical superiority of fresh arrangements, governments are not always in a strong position to introduce changes. A useful model of the political structure of the health care system distinguishes between three main interest groups: consumers; administrative rationalisers; and professional monopolists (Alford, 1975). The consumer is often the weakest and the professional monopolists are often the strongest. Standing behind the administrative rationalisers, governments are often obliged to approach health care reforms with caution. This is especially true when, as frequently happens, the consumers take side with the professional in opposing change.

References

Alford, R. (1975), *Health Care Politics*, Chicago, University of Chicago Press.

Barr, N. (1990), *Economic Theory and the Welfare State: A Survey and Reinterpretation*, Welfare State Programme, Discussion Paper No. 54, London School of Economics and Political Science.

Culyer, A. J. (1989), "The Normative Economics of Health Care Finance and Provision", *Oxford Review of Economic Policy*, Vol. 5, No. 1.

McPherson, K. (1990), "International Differences in Medical Care Practices", in *Health Care Systems in Transition*, OECD, Paris.

Payer, L. (1989), *Medicine and Culture*, London, Victor Gollancz.

Raffel, M. W. (1984), *Comparative Health Systems*, Pennsylvania State University.

Tussing, A. D. (1985), *Irish Medical Care Resources: An Economic Analysis*, The Economic and Social Research Institute, Dublin, Paper 126, November.

Williams, A. (1989), *Creating a Health Care Market: Ideology, Efficiency, Ethics and Clinical Freedom*, NHS White Paper Occasional Paper 5, University of York, March.

Chapter 2

SUB-SYSTEMS OF FINANCING AND DELIVERY OF HEALTH CARE

INTRODUCTION

At first sight, the seven countries in this study display great diversity in their methods of financing, organising and regulating health services. They differ in the extent to which they rely on out-of-pocket payments, private insurance, social insurance and general taxation for financing health services. They differ in the methods by which third parties pay providers. They differ in the extent to which the government itself has taken over the provision of health services or has left provision in private hands. And they differ in the extent to which regulation has been of the command and control type or has been devoted to promoting, as well as to channelling, market forces or quasi-market forces. These differences might appear to limit the usefulness of a comparative study of their health care reforms.

However, closer examination suggests that beneath this apparent diversity, the seven health care systems are made up from a short list of sub-systems of finance, payment and regulation, a few of which tend to dominate. A useful step towards understanding the national systems and their recent reforms is to differentiate these sub-systems, to identify the few which are dominant and to establish some hypotheses about their strengths and weaknesses against the objectives for health care which we discussed in the previous chapter.

The models suggested by Evans (1981) can be used to identify the sub-systems, and, indeed, to describe the whole health care systems of the seven countries later on. The models summarise alternative interactions between five principal sets of actors in health care systems: *a)* the consumers/patients; *b)* the first-level providers (such as general practitioners, or pharmacists supplying over the counter medicines); *c)* the second-level providers (such as most hospital services, and pharmacists who supply prescribed drugs); *d)* the insurers (or third-party payers); and *e)* the government in its capacity as regulator of the system. The main interactions between the five include: provision of services; referrals from first- to second-level providers; payment for services; payment for insurance; payment of insurance claims; and various forms of regulation by government. The models involve considerable simplification, but they help us to identify certain key building blocks which are found commonly across countries.

SUB-SYSTEMS OF SOURCES OF FINANCE AND METHODS OF PAYING PROVIDERS

It is convenient to start by looking at the main sub-systems of sources of finance and methods of paying providers, before bringing in varieties of government regulation. We can identify two major sources of finance: voluntary and compulsory (or public); and four major methods of paying providers: out-of-pocket by consumers, without insurance; out-of-pocket by consumers, who are reimbursed from insurance; indirectly by third parties, via arm's length contracts; and indirectly by third parties, via budgets and salaries within an integrated organisation. One of the resulting eight combinations of finance and payment – compulsory, out-of-pocket payment – is hardly found in practice. The remaining seven models are:

- The voluntary, out-of-pocket model;
- The voluntary reimbursement (of patients) model (to avoid confusion the term "reimbursement" is used only in the sense of reimbursement of patients in this book; this corresponds with British usage, and with French usage *remboursement*);
- The public reimbursement (of patients) model;
- The voluntary contract model;
- The public contract model;
- The voluntary integrated model; and
- The public integrated model.

These systems, and alternative methods of government regulation, are detailed below.

Certain other distinctions will be introduced which play a supporting role in this taxonomy. First, compulsory third-party payment systems divide into: those which are funded mainly by payroll contributions and are administered by quasi-autonomous sickness funds; and those which are funded mainly by general taxation and are administered by central or local government funding bodies. Second, methods of paying professionals divide into: fee for service (payment for each act); capitation (payments for each registered or enrolled client per period of time); and salary (payments for each period of time). The first two methods may be described as work-related, or as allowing "money to follow the patient" – this is truer for fee-for-service than for capitation. Third, methods of paying hospitals divide into: payment per case; payment per day; and prospective, global budgets. Again, the first two methods may be described as work-related or as allowing "money to follow the patient". Finally, health care providers divide into: independent professionals and institutions; and public employees and institutions. This last distinction, however, becomes blurred when it comes to salaried doctors who retain their professional autonomy.

The voluntary, out-of-pocket model

Chart 2.1 shows the simplest and earliest form of private, health care market without insurance but with direct, out-of-pocket, fee-for-service transactions between consumers (on the right) and first- and second-level providers, respectively (on the left). Solid lines show service flows, broken lines show financial flows and wavy lines show referral flows. First- and second-level providers are shown as multiple, to indicate that there is generally consumer-led competition between them (often subject to restrictions on advertising and on price competition and other restrictive practices). Chart 2.1 could also be used to depict cost-sharing under voluntary or compulsory health insurance, if it were blended with Charts 2.2-2.7 below.

Out-of-pocket payments depend on ability to pay. Where income is inadequate or where health expenditure is unexpected and catastrophic, the model will not be consistent with adequate or equitable access to health services or with adequate protection of income. Putting aside these distributional and risk issues, the achievement

Chart 2.1 **Voluntary, out-of-pocket payment for health care**

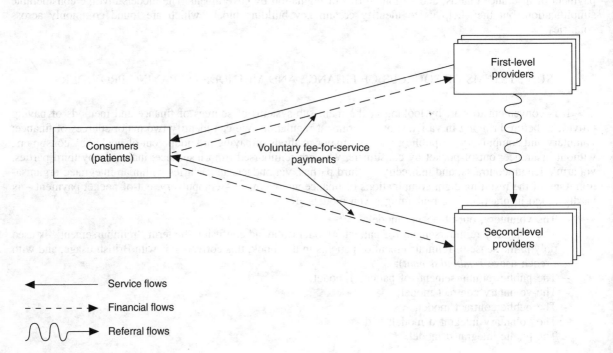

Service flows

Financial flows

Referral flows

of macro-economic and micro-economic efficiency is in doubt. Whereas consumers will be fully cost-conscious and will generally enjoy choice of provider, it is not clear that consumer sovereignty will prevail or that effective competition will take place. This is because of the asymmetry of knowledge between patients and physicians, and the possession of collective monopoly power by the latter. The model is likely to be most satisfactory for minor and routine health expenditure.

Given the prevalence of third-party payment for health services, the out-of-pocket model now plays only a supporting role in the health care systems described in this report. It is universally used for over-the-counter medicines, and for cost-sharing, especially for prescribed medicines. Private medical care consultations are often paid for out-of-pocket. In Ireland, over half of the population normally pays for general practitioner consultations out-of-pocket.

The voluntary reimbursement model

The working of private, medical care markets can be enhanced by the introduction of voluntary health insurance, but there tend to be unwanted side effects. Chart 2.2 shows ''conventional'' voluntary insurance of the indemnity kind, which involves reimbursement of patients for medical care bills, in part or in whole, and minimal interference with doctor/patient transactions of the kind described in Chart 2.1. There are: direct, fee-for-service payments to providers by consumers; competitive insurers; risk-related premiums; no connection between insurers and providers; and reimbursement of patients by insurers for medical bills covered under their insurance policies. There may well be cost-sharing between the patients and the insurers. A distinction can be made, within the consumers' box in the diagram, between the population which pays premiums and the consumers/patients who utilise services.

The voluntary reimbursement model will improve upon the out-of-pocket model to the extent that consumers can pool risks for unexpected medical care bills. There will be gains in welfare if individuals can exchange a certain premium for the uncertain prospect of either a higher income (if they remain healthy) or a financial loss (if they become sick and incur medical bills). However, these gains are eroded by administration costs which typically require 10 % to be added to the cost of actuarially fair premiums. Two other important drawbacks are associated with these arrangements.

Chart 2.2 **Voluntary insurance with reimbursement of patients**

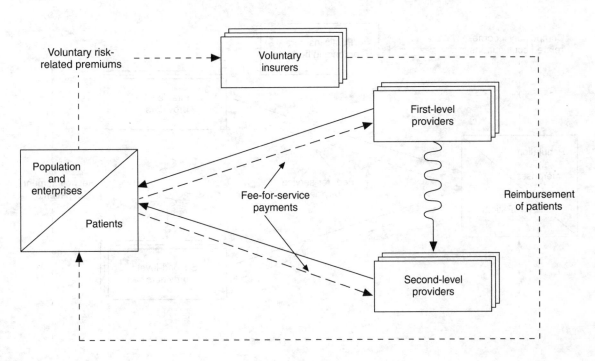

21

First, when the consumer is protected by this and other types of insurance, he or she has no incentive to restrain his or her demand (moral hazard) and knowing this, and with fee-for-service payments, the providers have positive incentives to induce demand. Competition may serve to stimulate the volume and quality of services and to raise, rather than to reduce, prices. For this reason, the reimbursement model is usually accompanied by cost-sharing. The tendency to encourage overspending will be reinforced if well-meaning governments have established tax relief for health insurance premiums.

The second major drawback is that nothing will be done to tackle systematic inequities. Access to insurance will be in accordance with ability to pay. Profit-maximising, competitive insurers have an incentive to select against poor risks or to load premiums against them. Individuals with pre-existing conditions are likely to be refused insurance altogether for these conditions. If health care prices are raised by the workings of reimbursement insurance, low-income groups may be made worse off.

Although this model has been described as "conventional" in deference to American literature, it was comparatively rare in Europe before public health insurance schemes were introduced. Rather, the dominant voluntary insurance models were of the contract or integrated type which provided benefits in kind – forerunners of health maintenance organisations (see below). Nevertheless, the reimbursement model often found a role after public schemes were set up. Arrangements approximating this model are now found in the private sectors in the United Kingdom and the Netherlands.

The public reimbursement model

The equity and risk selection problems of voluntary health insurance can be countered by public insurance with compulsory risk pooling, income-related contributions and subsidisation of contributions for the poor ("solidarity"). Chart 2.3 shows public insurance based on the same reimbursement principles explored above, with: direct, fee-for-service payment of providers by patients; compulsory, income-related contributions; non-competing sickness funds or funding bodies; no connections between sickness funds and providers; and reimbursement of patients by sickness funds for medical care bills according to the benefits of the scheme. There may well be cost-sharing between the patients and the insurers. Although there can be multiple sickness funds for different occupations, industries or localities, and even consumer choice between funds, there must be uniform

Chart 2.3 **Compulsory insurance with reimbursement of patients**

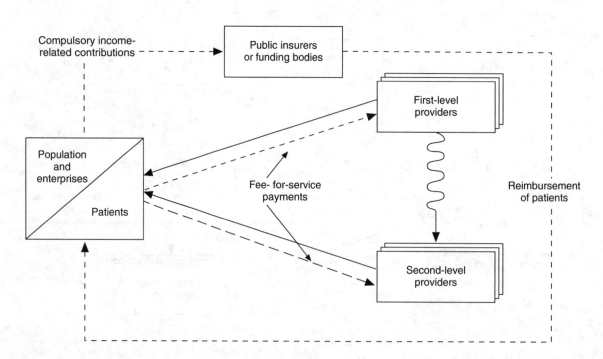

contribution rates and cross subsidies between funds if solidarity is to be preserved. For this reason, sickness funds are not shown as multiple. However, there can be consumer-led choice between providers.

This model can be designed to achieve a desired level of equity in access to and payment for services at the cost of compulsory contributions. Otherwise, it tends to share the defects of its private sector equivalent – moral hazard, supplier-induced demand and a tendency towards high administrative costs. Again, moral hazard can be countered by compulsory cost-sharing (such as the *ticket modérateur* in France).

The French system in the 1950s resembled this model in some respects, although the State subsequently stepped in behind the sickness funds to negotiate fees centrally with the doctors and other independent providers. Both the Belgian and French social health insurance systems retain elements of the public reimbursement model.

The voluntary contract model

Private markets in Europe long ago developed voluntary health insurance arrangements which involved contractual relationships between insurers and independent providers which enabled these providers (but not others) to supply services wholly or mainly free of charge to insured members (Green, 1985 and Abel Smith, 1988). These were forerunners of those health maintenance organisations in the United States which contract with individual physicians or with groups of physicians. Chart 2.4 shows such a model, with services provided in kind to patients, competition among insurers, community-rated (flat-rate) premiums and direct fee-for-service payments or capitation payments from the third parties to the providers. Providers are shown as multiple using dotted lines, to draw attention to the fact that competition is led by the insurers rather than by individual consumers.

This model comes in various versions: the insurers may be controlled by consumers (as in the early European friendly societies); they may be controlled by doctors or other providers (as in contemporary Individual Practice Associations in the United States); or they may be controlled by private organisations which are independent of both consumers and doctors. The benefits of the scheme may cover primary care only, or they may cover both primary and hospital care. Two important features of this model are: that consumer choice is generally restricted to the contracted providers; and that the insurers have both the incentive and the means to

Chart 2.4 **Voluntary insurance with insurer/provider contracts**

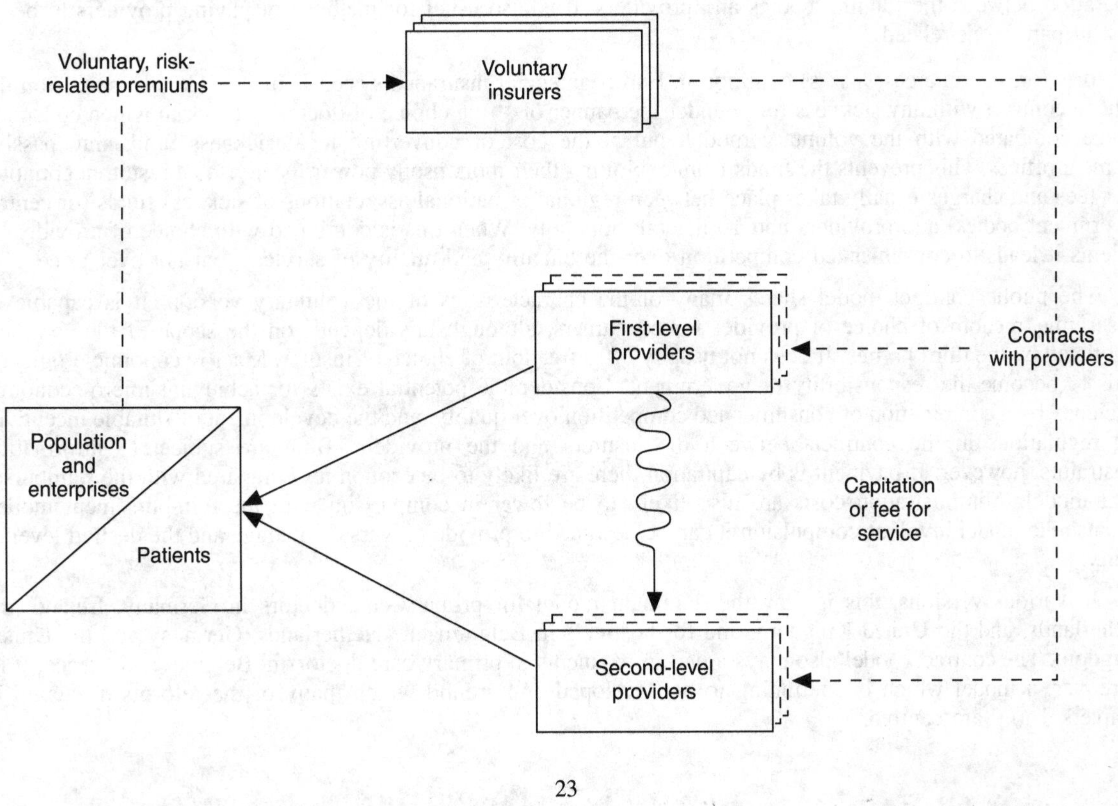

negotiate economical but high-quality care on behalf of consumers. If hospital care is offered under this model, primary care physicians are likely to act as gatekeepers.

Voluntary health insurance arrangements have a better potential for achieving macro- and micro-economic efficiency than "conventional" insurance. This is because of the countervailing power exercised by the insurers and the gatekeeper role played by the primary care physicians. In the hands of doctors, with fee-for-service payment, this potential may not be fully realised (Enthoven, 1988). Historical research in the United Kingdom (Green, 1985) as well as contemporary research in the United States (Enthoven, 1988), however, suggests that in the hands of consumers or independent insurers, and with capitation payments to doctors, this model can yield major savings without loss of quality. There are likely to be savings in administration costs over conventional insurance. The main disadvantage is the limited capacity to achieve equity or solidarity.

Although friendly societies played an important historical role in Europe, their markets tended to be confined to employed workers and their dependants. This left significant sections of the population without insurance. Friendly societies were also unpopular with organised medicine because of: the local market power which they gave to collectives of consumers; the threat of lay control which this posed for doctors; and their potential for eroding the size of the fee-for-service sector. They were swept aside in favour of: compulsory sickness funds; fee-for-service remuneration or central negotiation of capitation payments; and "free choice of doctor" when national schemes were introduced (Green, 1985; Abel-Smith, 1988). Abel Smith has suggested that the abolition of competition which resulted was the price that governments often found themselves paying in order to secure universal health insurance. Nevertheless, organisations of the Individual Practice Association and prepaid group practice type remain common in the Spanish private sector.

The public contract model

The basic design of the contract model was frequently imported into compulsory health insurance schemes in Europe. Chart 2.5 shows a public contract model with: services supplied to eligible consumers in kind; non-competing sickness funds or funding bodies; compulsory, income-related contributions; and direct fee-for-service or capitation payments by the sickness funds to independent providers. Again, this model comes in a number of versions. The source of funds may be general taxation rather than contributions. Instead of sickness funds, the third parties may be central or local government, or even first-level doctors in the case of second-level providers. And the providers, especially if they are hospitals, may be public bodies. The main features of this model are that the third parties are public and that they have contractual relations with the providers – in other words, there is separation between the funding bodies and providers. It is also usual for methods of paying providers to be, at least in part, work-related.

It is (or, in some cases, was) common in European social insurance systems for providers to have won the right to contract with any sickness fund, under the banner of "free choice of doctor". This can widen consumer choice compared with the voluntary model, but at the cost of converting local sickness funds into passive payment offices. This prevents the funds from exploiting their monopsony power locally. As a result, negotiation over fees and charges usually takes place between regional or national associations of sickness funds (or central government bodies) and providers under bilateral monopoly. When this is combined with choice of provider by patients it leads to consumer-led competition over the quantity and quality of services, but not over price.

The public contract model shares many of the characteristics of the voluntary version. It is capable of preserving freedom of choice of provider for consumers, although this depends on the scope of the contracts negotiated by the third parties. It does not usually offer freedom of choice of insurer. Macro-economic efficiency tends to become the responsibility of government. Considerable potential exists for achieving micro-economic efficiency by a combination of consumer-led competition over quality, and the development of suitable incentives and regulations in the contracts between the insurers and the providers. Both are subject to information constraints, however. If payment is by capitation there are likely to be economies compared with the reimbursement model. Administration costs are also likely to be lower in comparison with the reimbursement model. Because the model involves compulsion it can be designed to provide universal coverage and the desired level of equity.

In various versions, this is now the dominant model for primary care doctors in Germany, Ireland, the Netherlands, and the United Kingdom, and for hospitals in Belgium, the Netherlands, Germany and the United Kingdom. The contract model also plays a part in payments to primary care doctors in Belgium and France. It is, moreover, a model which is continuing to be developed and around which many of the reforms discussed in Chapters 3 to 9 are centred.

Chart 2.5 **Compulsory insurance with insurer/provider contracts**

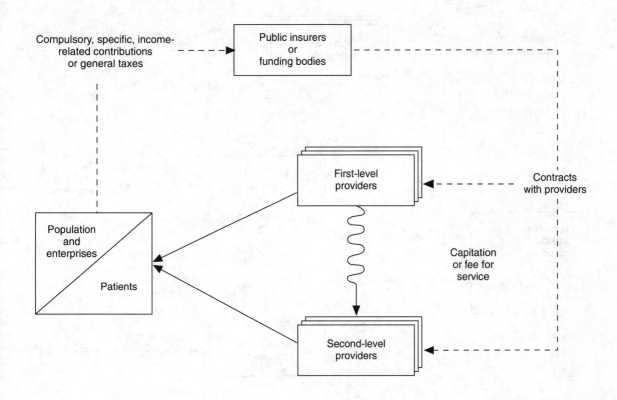

The voluntary integrated model

An early development in European private markets for medical care was that some groups of consumers as well as some insurers found it preferable to employ doctors on salary and to own their premises for primary care – and even hospital services – rather than to contract with independent providers. Later, these types of arrangements were rediscovered in the United States in what became known as the staff model of the health maintenance organisation. Chart 2.6 depicts the voluntary version of this model with: services supplied to patients in kind; competing insurers; voluntary, community-rated premiums; and vertical integration between the insurers and the providers, with salary and prospective budget payments to providers. Once again, providers are shown as multiple using dotted lines to indicate that consumers' choice of provider will follow, but be restricted by, their choice of insurer.

The voluntary integrated model preserves freedom of choice of insurer at the cost of restrictions on choice of provider. It restricts the managerial autonomy of doctors, although it can coexist with clinical autonomy. It possesses good potential for achieving macro- and micro-economic efficiency because there are: competitive incentives; good opportunities for managing the provision of care (through gatekeepers and the employment contract); and prospects for making administrative savings because of vertical integration. Although there are incentives towards under-service, these are counter-balanced by the need for the insurer to attract and hold the consumer in a competitive insurance market. However, as with the voluntary reimbursement and contract models, this model is unlikely to achieve the desired level of income protection or equity for vulnerable groups. This is because the acquisition of insurance will depend on ability to pay and there will be incentives for risk selection in a competitive market. The model was not popular with organised medicine in Europe and, in its voluntary form, failed to survive the establishment of compulsory national insurance schemes (Abel-Smith, 1988).

148,972

Chart 2.6 **Voluntary insurance with integration between insurers and providers**

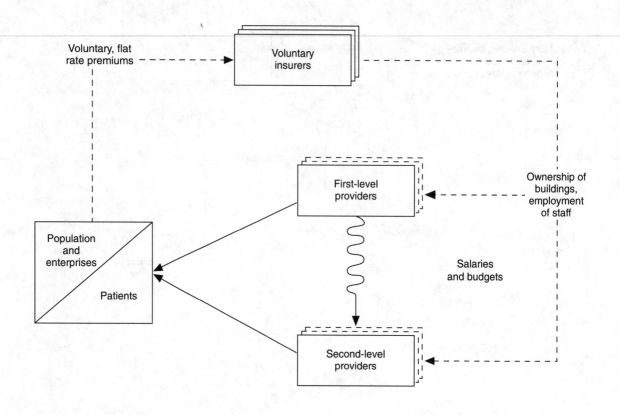

The public integrated model

The public version of the model discussed above was, however, widely adopted in compulsory systems. Chart 2.7 shows this version with: services supplied to patients in kind; third-party payments organised by public funding bodies, usually central or local government; financing by compulsory income-related contributions, often via general taxation; and payments to providers by salary and prospective budgets. Here, government is both the principal insurer and the major provider – as in the U.S. Department of Veterans Affairs. Variations on the model are possible, including financing by social insurance contributions and a greater or lesser degree of clinical autonomy. In general, consumers have no choice of insurer within the public scheme. In the pure version of the model, their choice of provider is also likely to be limited. However, even when consumer choice of provider is encouraged, it is likely to be financially ineffective (see below).

The public version of the integrated model is distinguished by lacking both consumer choice of insurer and choice (or effective choice) of provider. Compared with the voluntary version of the integrated model, the incentives for under-service are not countered by the need for the third parties to retain the custom of the insured. Compared with the public contract model, consumer choice of provider and choice of hospital by the primary care doctor – although these may exist – are ineffective. Money does not follow the patient when providers are paid by salaries and global budgets. This means that the incentives for providers are perverse (Enthoven, 1985). Efficient providers are rewarded by more work but not by increased resources. Inefficient providers are rewarded by a quiet life and idle resources. Queues for services are commonplace, and patients tend to become grateful supplicants rather than empowered consumers. In addition, it lacks incentives for providers to minimise unit costs. For example, underspending by hospitals in one year is often met by grant reductions in the following year. Macro-economic efficiency becomes the responsibility of government, and because of the integrated nature of the model it is relatively easy for the government to control total health expenditure at the level it desires. The integrated model is probably capable of achieving further administrative economies compared with the contract

Chart 2.7 Compulsory insurance with integration between insurance and provision

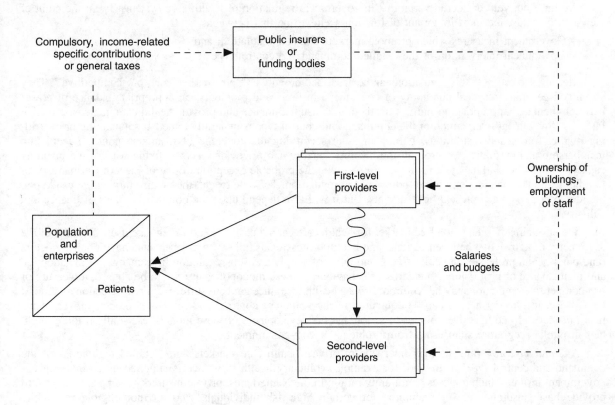

model. Because it involves compulsion this model is capable of achieving universal coverage and the desired level of equity.

This is the dominant model in Spain and for public hospitals in France and in Ireland. It was, until recently, the model used for public hospitals in the United Kingdom. A totalitarian version was virtually the sole model in Eastern Germany before reunification.

Mixed systems

As we will see in Chapters 3 to 9, the seven countries all have health care systems which are mixtures of several of these seven sub-systems of financing and delivery of health care. There are good reasons for this. Voluntary payment systems can act as safety valves for compulsory systems. Moderate cost-sharing can mitigate the adverse incentive effects of generous third-party coverage, particularly in the reimbursement model (van de Ven, 1983). The public contract model has been popular for ambulatory medical care, presumably because it helps to preserve the independence of doctors. The public integrated model has been popular for hospital care, partly because it favours control of costs. However, all of the national systems are dominated by just one or two of the sub-systems.

First, the voluntary models have come to play a minor or supplementary role in all of these countries except the Netherlands, where the private reimbursement model still played an important part at the end of the 1980s. Second, among the compulsory models, the public contract and public integrated models are dominant, complemented by, at most, minor cost-sharing. Although Belgium and France still rely upon the public reimbursement model to some extent, this has been blended with the public contract model or, in the case of public hospitals in France, overridden by the integrated model. Germany, the Netherlands and, more recently, the United Kingdom, rely mainly on the public contract model. Spain relies mainly on the integrated model. Ireland relies on a mixture of the two.

VARIETIES OF GOVERNMENT REGULATION

We have not yet considered variations in government regulation of health care systems. From the point of view of this study, the most important distinction seems to be that between:

- Government measures which promote markets and self-regulation; and
- Government intervention of the detailed command-and-control type.

Measures to promote self-regulation can be described broadly as ''pro-market'' or ''pro-competitive''. They are aimed generally at: local autonomy of consumers, insurers and providers, an appropriate balance of power between them and appropriate incentives for them to consume, finance and provide health care in a cost-effective fashion. Government intervention of the command-and-control type is generally aimed at supplanting or overriding market forces and institutions. It may include: specifying the coverage of insurance policies, regulating membership and premiums, controlling the quantity, quality and prices of services, fixing wages, and planning capacity. In practice, all the systems in this study – with the probable exception of that of Eastern Germany, prior to reunification – contain a mixture of both types of regulation. To some extent, the precise mix will depend upon the ideology of past and present governments. But it will also depend upon the dominant models of finance and delivery.

We have already seen that a free market for health care cannot easily be left to regulate itself. Because of the asymmetry of knowledge between patients and health professionals, all seven governments have granted doctors (and other health professionals) collective monopolies of supply and self-regulation in exchange for the adoption and maintenance of professional standards of behaviour. If these monopolies are not to be abused, a measure of pro-competitive regulation may be required. Private health insurance tends to suffer from risk selection and moral hazard. Because moral hazard can be countered in the voluntary contract and integrated models, governments may introduce pro-competitive policies to encourage the development of these models, especially if these might benefit public programmes suffering from problems of cost-containment.

Alternatively, governments may intervene in private health care markets with detailed regulations of the command-and-control type. In Ireland, for example, voluntary health insurance is supplied by a single, quasi-government insurer which imposes community rating. In the Netherlands, private insurers have been mandated to provide basic insurance at set premiums for certain high-risk individuals who are not eligible for public insurance. In the United Kingdom, however, where private health insurance plays a strictly supplementary role, there is relatively little regulation of the private insurance market.

Where governments have introduced public financing, they have generally gained control of the corresponding health insurance function – more so in the case of centrally financed schemes than in the case of quasi-independent sickness funds. Despite this, the public reimbursement model, at least in its pure form, is likely to suffer from problems of cost-containment because of its lack of influence over providers. This may lead to detailed government regulation by the backdoor of, say, the capacity of providers and the prices which they are allowed to charge.

The public contract model is less vulnerable to cost-containment problems and is much more amenable to local self-regulation, especially if the insurers are allowed to exert monopsony power, if money follows the patient, and if competition is encouraged between providers. Germany provides an example of this. The integrated model brings with it government control over both insurers and providers – typically through line management. Paradoxically, this model can coexist with higher levels of clinical autonomy than other models (Schulz and Harrison, 1986) and considerable delegation to local management bodies. This is because of its ability to secure a firm framework of expenditure control.

SUMMARY OF HYPOTHESES ABOUT THE PERFORMANCE OF SUB-SYSTEMS

In this chapter, we have made preliminary assessments of the sub-systems of finance, payment and regulation of health care, in the light of the policy objectives which we discussed in the previous chapter. This provides us with some hypotheses about the performance of the sub-systems, to be kept in mind when we examine whole systems and their reforms in Chapters 3 to 9.

Three main pointers emerge: all the voluntary models have difficulties meeting adequacy and distributional objectives; both types of reimbursement model have difficulties achieving the cost-containment objective; and there are question marks against the ability of the public integrated model to achieve micro-economic objectives. The public contract model has been granted the highest positive score among the seven sub-systems. Question marks are placed against the health outcome objective for all the models. This is because there is scant evidence

28

that any one model performs better than any other in this respect. Uncertainty about health outcome is an obstacle which all governments face in their attempts to improving the performance of their health care systems.

References

Abel-Smith, B. (1988), "The Rise and Decline of the Early HMOs: Some International Experiences", *The Milbank Quarterly*, Vol. 66, No. 4.

Evans, R. G. (1981), "Incomplete Vertical Integration: the Distinctive Structure of the Health-Care Industry", in J. van der Gaag and M. Perlman (editors), *Health, Economics and Health Economics*, Amsterdam.

Enthoven, A. C. (1985), *Reflections on the Management of the National Health Service*, Nuffield Provincial Hospitals Trust, London.

Enthoven, A. C. (1988), *Theory and Practice of Managed Competition in Health Care Finance*, Amsterdam.

Green, D. G. (1985), *Working Class Patients and the Medical Establishment*, Gower.

Schulz, R. and Harrison, S. (1986), "Physician Autonomy in the Federal Republic of Germany, Great Britain and the United States", *International Journal of Health Planning and Management*, Vol. 2.

van de Ven, W. P. M. M. (1983), *Effects of Cost-Sharing in Health Care*, Effective Health Care, Vol. 1, No. 1.

Chapter 3

THE REFORM OF THE HEALTH SYSTEM IN BELGIUM[1]

INTRODUCTION

The Belgian health care system, like that of France, can be described as a marriage between national health insurance and independent medical practice or *médecine libérale*. Compulsory health insurance covers major risks for the whole population and minor as well as major risks for 85 % of the population. Five *mutualités* (private non-profit sickness funds or friendly societies) and a single public fund act as carrriers of insurance cover. There is free choice of doctor and most of the providers are independent and paid by fee for service. The first part of this chapter describes the organisation and financing of the system.

Although there have been no sudden structural reforms to the health care system over the past decade, the government introduced a number of important alterations to the system during the 1980s. In the main, these were aimed at controlling the growth of health expenditure. The chapter discusses the background to these reforms, including dfficulties with cost-containment and the raising of revenues, as well as structural weaknesses in the health care system itself. Some of the main changes are then outlined.

The chapter goes on to consider some evidence on the growth and performance of the system, both in relation to the government's policy aims for health and when compared with the other six countries in this study.

Two main issues continue to dominate the health policy debate within Belgium: how to control the cost of health care within the context of health insurance; and the question of who will pay for the higher cost of health care. The chapter concludes by discussing a recent cost-containment reform which may provide the best opportunity for preserving, in the long term, the benefits which *la médecine libérale* can bring.

HEALTH CARE SYSTEM DESCRIBED

In terms of the models set out in Chapter 2, the Belgian health care system is a blend of the public reimbursement and the public contract models. Patients pay for most ambulatory care and are partially reimbursed by the *mutualités*. The bulk of hospital costs, however, is paid directly to the hospitals by the *mutualités*. Most health service professionals are in independent practice and there is a mix of private and public hospitals. The system is regulated by a mixture of government regulation (central and regional) and self-regulation by the insurers and providers. The way in which the system is administered reflects the fact that the country is culturally and linguistically heterogeneous, being divided between Dutch-speaking Flanders and French-speaking Wallonia and Brussels, each with some regional autonomy.

Chart 3.1 is a simplified depiction of the organisation and financing of the system. At the bottom left of the diagram is the population, most of whom become patients in any one year. At the bottom right are the, mainly independent, providers. At the top of the diagram are the third-party payers. Service flows are shown as solid lines and financing flows as broken lines.

The providers have been divided into: public health services; independent pharmacists; independent professionals providing ambulatory care; private, non-profit hospitals, public hospitals; and rest and nursing homes. In addition, there are homes for the elderly and domiciliary support services; these are only partially funded by health insurance and are not shown in the diagram. The third-party payers have been divided into: the *mutualités* in their role of carriers of compulsory insurance; the *mutualités* in their role as suppliers of supplementary insurance; and the private insurance companies.

Total payments to providers were BF 417 billion in 1987, of which 36 % was met by social security contributions, 39 % was met out of general taxation, 10 % represented a social security deficit and other payments to social security, 3 % was met by voluntary health insurance and 12 % by out-of-pocket payments. About two

Chart 3.1 **Key relationships in the Belgian health care system in 1987**
(billions BF)

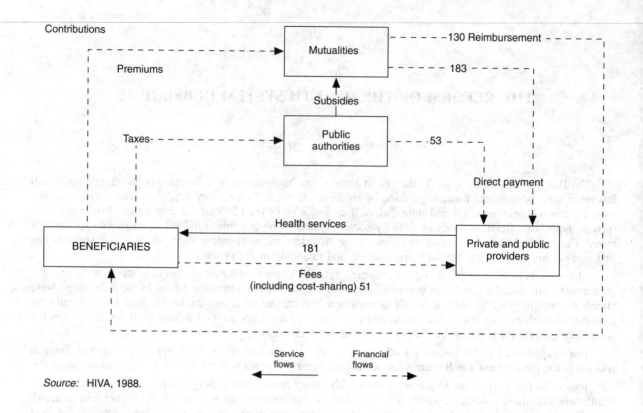

Source: HIVA, 1988.

thirds of the 88 % of total expenditure which was met by insurers represented direct payments to providers and about one-third took the form of reimbursement of bills paid by patients (Wouters *et al.,* 1988).[2]

RELATIONSHIP BETWEEN PATIENTS AND PROVIDERS

Ambulatory medical care

Both general practitioners and specialists are independent professionals, paid by fee for service. They usually operate from single-handed practices, often based in their homes and, in the case of specialists, from hospital out-patient departments. The patient is free to approach either a general practitioner (GP) or a specialist for a primary consultation. Specialists do not receive a reduced fee for a primary consultation. Partly because the physician/population ratio is high, ambulatory medical care is highly competitive and doctors seem to be very responsive to patients. GPs do more home visits than office consultations. Patients seldom wait more than a few hours after calling a GP by telephone (Nys and Quaethoven, 1984). However, "medical ethics" means that there is very little price competition, at least among GPs (Nonneman, 1990).

The patient pays by fee for service (BF 425 for a GP consultation, BF 558 for a home visit and BF 713 for a typical specialist consultation in 1989) according to a fee schedule established between the representatives of the medical profession and the *mutualités,* and is partially reimbursed by his or her *mutualité* on submission of the bill. In the case of GPs, the fees are lower for a doctor who has not been retrained. For most medical consultations, the patient pays co-insurance of 25 %, while widows, disabled, old age pensioners and orphans (VIPOs) with an annual income of less than BF 356 113 in 1989 in the case of a household pay on average 10 %. Some doctors have not accepted the negotiated fee schedule and, in certain circumstances, are free to extra bill. These doctors have to advertise their lack of affiliation. However, because there are affiliated physicians in all areas, this does not pose problems for the poor.

Chart 3.2 Detail of relationships in the Belgian health care system in 1989

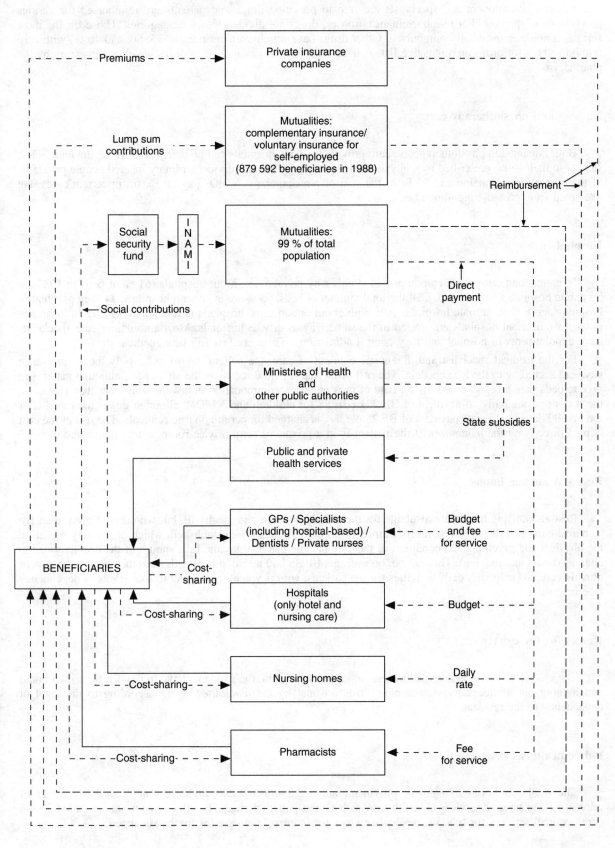

Pharmaceuticals

General practitioners and specialists are free to prescribe drugs and patients are reimbursed for various proportions of the cost. For reimbursement purposes, drugs are divided into six categories. Those for the most serious conditions are wholly reimbursed. Other drugs have reimbursement rates of 75, 50, and 40 %, with zero reimbursement for drugs on a negative list. A lump-sum payment is applied to drugs which are made up by the pharmacist.

Nursing and physiotherapy care

Both nursing and physiotherapeutic care provided outside hospitals can be partly paid for by the *mutualités,* subject to their being prescribed by a physician. Payment is by fee for service. Ordinary insured people pay 25 % of the cost of home nursing and 40 % of the cost of physiotherapy. VIPOs pay 20 %, or, in certain cases, are exempted from cost-sharing altogether.

Hospital care

In-patient and out-patient care is provided either by private, non-profit hospitals (61 % of beds in 1987) or by public hospitals (39 % of beds). Of the total number of beds, 68 % are in general hospitals, 24 % in psychiatric hospitals and 8 % in chronic hospitals. Although about one in three hospitals is municipal, for health insurance purposes municipal hospitals are treated in the same way as private hospitals. Most ambulatory care specialists have appointments in hospital and they control admissions. There are few full-time medical staff.

For the medical specialist and diagnostic element of care, the patient has to make only the co-insurance payment according to the fee schedule. The rest of the fee is paid directly by the *mutualités,* although patients in private beds may be extra billed. In the case of nursing and accommodation in a ward with more than two beds, the patient pays a daily co-payment of BF 221 (BF 88 for children and VIPOs), although this is increased after the first 90 days. A separate payment of BF 25 per day is charged for certain pharmaceuticals. The rest of the cost is paid directly by the *mutualités.* If the patient is in a private or semi-private room, extra charges are due.

Rest and nursing homes

Rest and nursing homes are available for the elderly who are chronically ill, but who do not need intensive technical care. In 1983, new criteria for admission to these homes were established, which are closely related to the physical and psychological condition of the patient. The patients pay the full amount of the accommodation charges (board and lodging). This can be, on average, BF 35 000 per month. Health insurance covers the cost of nursing care and help with daily activities for the patients, with payments according to four levels of dependency (see below).

Homes for the elderly

The elderly can also be admitted to residential homes. Again, the residents have to pay for their own board and lodging but, if necessary, any nursing costs are met by the *mutualités,* again according to the level of dependency of the resident.

Public health services

The public authorities (regional, provincial and local government) organise and finance a number of preventive and curative services in health care such as: out-patient perinatal health care, out-patient mental health care, medical services for schools, medical services for industry and care for the handicapped.

RELATIONSHIP BETWEEN POPULATION AND THIRD-PARTY PAYERS

Compulsory health insurance

Belgium has had a compulsory health insurance system since 1945. Administration of the system is divided between the five non-profit *mutualités* which had previously organised voluntary insurance, and one public fund. The *mutualités* are organised mainly according to religious or political affiliations. Membership of a fund is compulsory for most employees, self-employed and retired people, but the choice of the fund is free. Since the statutory insurance cover offered by the funds and the contribution rates levied by them are identical, the *mutualités* compete for new members only on supplementary services, on geographical convenience and on the speed of settling claims. Competition is fierce, nevertheless, partly because revenue for administration depends on the size of the membership. Because the remuneration levels and risks of their respective memberships vary considerably, the funds have different capacities to earn contributions, as well as different claims' experience. To preserve solidarity, surpluses and deficits are effectively pooled by the National Institute for Health, Sickness and Invalidity Insurance (INAMI).

The *mutualités* receive their funds from and are supervised by INAMI. This is administered by a general board made up of representatives of employers, of employees, of *mutualités,* of providers and of government. The government has a power of veto over decisions.

The benefits of the statutory scheme include both health insurance cover and income support in the event of illness. In the case of health insurance cover, two, financially separate, schemes operate: the *general scheme* covers both major and minor risks and applies to employees and civil servants, retired, handicapped and their dependants, making up 85 % of the population; the *scheme for the self-employed* covers only major risks and accounts for most of the remaining 15 % of the population. Major risks mainly involve in-patient care and special technical services. Minor risks include out-patient care, medicines, dental care, etc.

The two main sources of funding of compulsory health insurance are social security contributions (58 % of revenue in 1987) and state subsidies (42 % of revenue). Additional sources, such as contributions from old-age pensioners and taxes on car insurance, account for the remainder of the total revenue. The contribution to health insurance represents 2.55 % of the gross wages of the employees and 3.80 % for the employer, which results in a total contribution of 6.35 % (as at 1 January 1989) deducted from gross wages. There is no upper or lower income limit to the contributions for the employed. For the self-employed the contribution represents 3.20 % of their income, with an upper limit of an annual income of BF 2.1 million. Old-age pensioners pay a contribution of 2.55 % of their pension over a minimum level.

Voluntary health insurance

Besides compulsory health insurance, the *mutualités* organise voluntary health insurance for minor risks (out-patient care, medicines, dental care, etc.) for the self-employed, and complementary insurance to cover additional services for all of their affiliated members. About 70 % of the self-employed take out insurance for minor risks.

Although private health insurance is a relatively small part of the whole sector, it is currently experiencing a steady growth, especially for hospital costs. Private health insurance is offered by private, for-profit companies in Belgium. Turnover is estimated at BF 5.5 billion.

General taxation

General taxation accounts for 39 % of the cost of health services. Of this, about two-thirds represents the subsidy to the statutory health insurance scheme and about one-third payments for public health services.

RELATIONSHIP BETWEEN THIRD-PARTY PAYERS AND PROVIDERS

Ambulatory and hospital medical care

Fees for medical and technical services (for example, laboratory tests) for ambulatory patients are usually paid by the patient (subject to reimbursement). Fees for similar services for in-patients are usually paid by the *mutualités.* The fee schedule on which reimbursement or payment is based is negotiated each year between representatives of the *mutualités* and of the medical profession. The agreements must be approved by the government. These arrangements amount to a bilateral monopoly supervised by the government.

An agreement is not implemented if it is rejected by more than 40 % of practitioners. Three measures are then available to the government:

- Submit an alternative draft agreement to the practitioners;
- Impose fees for some or all of the services;
- Fix the reimbursement levels. The practitioners are then free to fix their own fees.

The fees which specialists earn from treating in-patients are usually shared between the hospital and the physicians, but practice on this is very variable.

Pharmaceuticals

The prices of all drugs marketed in Belgium are subject to product-by-product negotiation between the Ministry of Economic Affairs and the pharmaceutical companies. Further bargaining takes place between a committee of the INAMI and representatives of the pharmaceutical industry on the price of drugs approved for reimbursement.

Nursing and physiotherapy

Nurses and physiotherapists in ambulatory care are paid by fee for service. As with ambulatory and hospital medical care, the fee schedule is negotiated between the *mutualités* and representatives of the professions. The government has a power of veto, and the agreement must be accepted by 60 % of the professionals concerned before being made effective. Individual nurses or physiotherapists are free to reject the agreement and extra bill but, if they do so, the reimbursement rates to their patients are reduced by 25 %. Since April 1991, nurses have been paid on a daily rate basis, depending on the degree of dependency of their patients.

Hospital care

The *mutualités* finance directly the bulk of hospital operating costs. Until 1982, nursing and accommodation costs were paid at per diem rates assessed retrospectively. This gave hospitals incentives to expand costs and length of stay. Since 1982, budgets and targets for the annual number of days to be provided have been fixed prospectively by the government, but the *mutualités* still pay the hospitals for each day of stay for their members at the agreed daily rate. Hospitals which exceed their quota of days receive 30 % of the daily rate to cover variable costs. Hospitals which fail to reach their quota of days receive 50 % of the daily rate for the shortfall to cover their fixed costs. Hospital nurses and other hospital staff, apart from doctors, are salaried and their wages are negotiated centrally, with some scope for local variations.

In setting the budgets, an element of comparison with other hospitals is taken into account. Hospital costs are divided into three parts:

- Depreciation and other investment costs, which are paid at their actual level and are not index-linked;
- Hotel service costs, which are being brought into line with average costs in similar hospitals, are subject to index-linking;
- Nursing and medical supplies costs, which are gradually being adjusted according to specialty mix and the level of clinical activity.

The budgets are designed to contain overall costs. Because they standardize costs between similar hospitals – and are responsive, to some extent, to workload – the budgets also promote efficiency. However, budgets do not cover specialist medical fees, which are generally shared with the hospital. In practice, patient-day quotas have not been revised significantly since 1982 (Hermesse, 1986; De Cooman et Marchand, 1987).

As far as financing rules for hospital investments are concerned, private and public hospitals are treated in much the same way. Agreement, in principle, for construction or renovation work is granted by the regional Minister for Health. In the case of private hospitals, 60 % of investment costs, limited to a maximum amount per bed, is met through a capital grant by the regional government. The balance, or 40 %, is met out of government-backed loans and is paid off in 33 years for buildings, ten years for non-medical equipment and five years for medical equipment. This is achieved by including appropriate depreciation and interest charges in the budget, and hence in the daily price, paid by the *mutualités*. For public hospitals, the relevant percentages are 70 % and 30 %. Payments related to medical technical services not included in the daily price must be covered by medical fees.

Rest and nursing homes

The *mutualités* meet the cost of nursing care and help with daily activities. Since April 1991, daily rates have been tailored according to four categories of dependency and range from BF 50 to 1 300 per day.

Homes for the elderly

The *mutualités* meet the cost of nursing care and daily activities if residents are assessed as eligible for admission to rest and nursing homes. The daily rates are tailored to the same four categories of dependency as for rest and nursing homes but are lower, ranging from BF 35 to 840 per day.

GOVERNMENT PLANNING AND REGULATION

The Belgian health care system displays a mixture of direct planning and regulation by central and local government and self-government by the insurers and providers.

Central government takes the final responsibility for the scope of benefits, for the level of the contributions to the compulsory health insurance system, and for the conventions and agreements which govern the relationship between the *mutualités* and the providers. It plays a leading role in cost-containment by its detailed involvement in the setting of hospital budgets, its veto powers over the level of fees and its negotiating of drug prices. Central government also takes the lead in planning (and, in part, financing) investment in hospitals. It sets the accreditation standards which require that hospitals meet certain structural and architectural standards, department by department. In addition, central government is responsible for the accreditation of doctors and ancillary care providers. However, the policy on access to and graduation from medical school is non-interventionist. Controls operate only on training posts for hospital specialists.

In 1980, Belgium's constitutional structure underwent considerable change. Important functions were moved from the national government to the Dutch and French-speaking communities. Since then, the regional governments have been responsible for the application of hospital accreditation standards and planning measures and, in part, for the financing of hospital investment. Regional ministries are responsible for health education and preventive medicine.

Within this framework of central and local government regulation, considerable autonomy is granted to the consumers, third-party payers and the providers. Under the statutory health insurance scheme, consumers are free to choose both their insurer and their provider. The *mutualités*, which see themselves as representing the consumers, play an important role in bargaining with the medical and other independent professions on fees, and with the drug companies on pharmaceutical prices. Again, the negotiations resemble bilateral monopoly. The *mutualités* also take a lead in recommending changes in the level of cost-sharing by patients for services. The doctors themselves staff a committee (half appointed by INAMI) for investigating abnormal levels of service or prescribing by individual doctors.

BACKGROUND TO RECENT REFORMS

The Belgian health care system demonstrates many strengths. It offers comprehensive compulsory health insurance cover to 85 % of the population and compulsory cover for major risks to the remaining 15 % of the population. This ensures a high level of solidarity and equity in access. Patients enjoy greater freedom of choice of provider than in any of the other six countries in this study. Consumers are free to choose both their insurer and their provider. There is no GP gatekeeper. The system also gives providers a great deal of autonomy. Nearly all providers, including hospital specialists, are paid by fee for service. As a result, both ambulatory medical and hospital care are said to be very competitive (Nonneman, 1990). While by the very partial measure available, standards of health outcome seem to be no better than those of comparable countries, the system seems to be remarkably responsive to patients. Access to GP services seems to be particularly quick and convenient, and it is said that there are few people waiting for hospital in-patient care.

However, there are difficulties with both cost-containment and the raising of revenue, neither of which is surprising. Apart from the extra demands caused by an ageing population and the continuing development of expensive, new medical techniques, the system contains financial incentives which encourage the growth of expenditure. Consumers have little incentive to limit their demands, despite moderate cost-sharing for ambulatory care and token cost-sharing for hospital care. Moreover, most providers have every incentive (financially) to expand services and to induce demand because they are paid by fee for service. Although the *mutualités*, co-ordinated and backed by the government, asserted their bargaining power during the 1970s in setting fees and charges for their beneficiaries, the volume of services remained relatively uncontrolled. Health expenditure grew rapidly in the 1970s and, given Belgium's standard of living, is higher than would be expected.

In addition, there have been structural weaknesses. For example, the fee-for-service system seems to have favoured prescribing and laboratory testing rather than, for instance, prevention. Some commentators have pointed to excessive care of some types – for example, too many hospital beds – to a shortage of nursing home beds and to the disproportionately large numbers of small hospitals.

The system has also suffered from weaknesses in management arrangements. The juxtaposition of fee for service for specialists, with budgeting for nursing and accommodation costs, leads to tensions between doctors and managers. Furthermore, management information in hospitals is often inadequate.

REFORMS IN THE EIGHTIES

Raising revenue

High levels of unemployment in the early 1980s exacerbated the health system's difficulties on the revenue side. In response, the Minister for Social Affairs launched a special fund in 1982 to bring about short-term financial equilibrium in the social security system. The fund is supported by special contributions from wage earners and is not intended to form a permanent, new structural element in the financing of social security. The more fundamental weaknesses in the financing of the social security system (which arise from the deteriorating ratio of contributors to beneficiaries) were partly dealt with by a government decision at the end of 1983 to increase the rate of contributions to the health care insurance system by 0.75 to 6.35 % of gross wages. Old-age pensioners with a pension above a certain level have had to pay a 2.55 % contribution since 1981. This contribution, however, only finances 4 % of the consumption of the retired population.

Curbing expenditure and dealing with structural problems

Ambulatory care

Since 1979, a system of profiles has progressively been established for each prescribing doctor and for paramedicals such as physiotherapists. The profiles are analysed by committees and can give rise to sanctions or further investigation in the event of outliers. In 1990, the whole procedure for revising examinations and selecting profiles was altered in order to speed up the procedure of selection and sanctions. Sanctions may be applied by *mutualités*, and referrals withheld from certain doctors. Committees are also organised on a provincial level so as to speed up the process of examining profiles related to local practices.

Pharmaceuticals

A new reimbursement system for medicines, prepared by the *mutualités*, was introduced at the end of 1980. The new system introduced cost-sharing proportional to the price of the medicine; the co-insurance rate was made higher for less vital medicines. This meant a complete change from the old system where there was no relation between the price of the medicine and the charge to the patient.

More recently, the government decided to strike off the list of reimbursable drugs as many as 163 industrially produced medicines. At the same time, the reimbursement rate of many medicines (peripheral and cerebral vasodilatoral drugs, in particular) was lowered, especially those whose medical usefulness was questioned. It was anticipated that these two measures would reduce the annual rate of increase of the drugs bill by about one-fifth. The government has also tried to encourage the production and consumption of generic medicines, which, on average, are 10 to 15 % cheaper than the brand name drugs. So far, however, these measures have not had any success. A transparency committee was set up in 1990 to examine whether the prices of medicines correspond to their therapeutic value per unit. A positive list has also been introduced for drugs made up by pharmacists.

Financing and restructuring hospitals

In 1982, the government announced reforms in the hospital sector which included: the introduction of prospective global budgets; reduction in the number of beds; the substitution of beds in rest and nursing homes for those in acute hospitals; and the closure or merger of small hospitals.

The introduction of global budgets had various aspects. First, a budget was fixed for each hospital. Second, a quota of days was fixed for each. Days in excess of this quota were paid at a rate which reflected variable costs. Any shortfall in actual days was paid at a rate which reflected fixed costs only. In addition, moves towards standardizing budgets across hospitals in accordance with case-mix and structural criteria were gradually developed. Finally, plans are now in place to use the budgets to provide incentives for the pursuit of quality assurance and medical audits.

The reduction in the number of hospital beds involved a moratorium, which prevented the number of hospital beds from exceeding the maximum number reached on 1 July 1982. No new hospital can be opened without the closure of an equivalent one. In addition, financial incentives were introduced for closing or converting beds (see below). Between 1982 and 1989, this resulted in a 14 % decrease in the number of acute hospital beds, half of the target.

Restructuring hospitals involved the establishment of specialised hospital geriatric services (G services) and the introduction of a conversion system whereby acute and chronic beds can be converted to G beds or to beds in rest and nursing homes (both in hospitals and rest homes). This was designed to produce savings because admissions to rest and nursing homes are reimbursed at a lower rate than admissions to general hospitals. At the end of 1989, nearly 18 000 places had been created in rest and nursing homes as a result of the closure of wards in acute hospitals. Nevertheless, this policy is not complete as there are still nearly 4 000 V beds (beds for patients with long-term illnesses) which have not yet been converted. The fate of these beds is the subject of a political debate.

The concentration of hospitals involved setting the accreditation standard at a minimum of 150 beds with appropriate staff and services. In the event of hospitals failing to fulfil these conditions, mergers or closures are required.

Further steps were taken recently to close beds and to economise on investment. First, if investments lead to a net reduction in beds of 25 % or more, regional governments are allowed to decrease their contribution from 60 % to 30 %, leaving the *mutualités* to bear the remainder of the cost. As a result, regional governments are giving priority to construction projects which reduce beds. Second, the National Minister for Health fixed a ceiling for the increase of the investment budget at about 5 % per year. Regional governments cannot sanction construction projects whose aggregate costs would exceed this ceiling.

Hospital management and management information

In 1986, a law on hospitals dealt with the relationship between hospital managers and doctors. It proposed:
– The appointment of a chief doctor to assist in the direction of the hospital;
– The compulsory creation of a medical council in each hospital with a specified advisory role;
– The creation of a permanent committee for consultations between the managers and the medical staff; and
– The establishment of the principle of mandatory central billing for medical fees.

Since 1983, the system for the collection and transmission of hospital management data has been greatly improved and has been computerised. Since 1985, hospitals have been obliged to deal with insurance companies by means of magnetic tapes, and pathology laboratories must do the same. Nevertheless, the computer system is not complete, as there are no data yet available on the diagnoses of in-patients. To remedy this, all hospitals have been required since October 1990 to keep improved in-patient records to include: the principal and secondary diagnosis of the in-patient; data from the invoice department of the hospital; and the type of medical care provided. These should provide the basis for an analysis of patients and costs by diagnosis-related groups. The new information system offers many possibilities including: epidemiological studies, hospital planning, accreditation standards, as well as improvements in internal and external financing techniques.

Financing laboratory testing

Up to 1988, laboratory testing was mainly financed on a fee-for-service basis at an average rate for all costs incurred, both fixed and variable. This system encouraged over-production. In 1985, within the framework of the agreement concluded between medical doctors and *mutualités,* the Minister for Health established a national budget. However, the reimbursement of laboratory testing remained on a fee-for-service basis and there was no incentive for individual providers to change their behaviour. The only sanction for exceeding the national budget was a further reduction of rates (such as by 30 % in August 1988). From 1 August 1988, the first steps were taken towards a new system which bases payment on admissions for in-patients and items of service for ambulatory patients.

In 1989, the Minister again fixed a national budget for laboratory testing and introduced further new financing methods. The law now stipulates that each laboratory should repay a certain percentage, depending on its size, if the out-patient budget is exceeded. For in-patients, payment per test is mostly replaced by payment per day, in addition to a payment per admission. The daily rates were calculated on an historic basis and varied enormously between hospitals. In 1990 and 1991, steps were taken to correct these historic rates, taking into account the case-mix in the hospitals.

The same techniques were introduced in 1989 to cover the costs of hospital pharmacies. Their extension to radiology services was being considered in 1990.

Psychiatric care

In 1990, the government decided to implement new policies for psychiatric services:
- A further reduction in the number of beds for long-term hospital care. Psychiatric hospital wards will be converted into psychiatric nursing homes. The psychiatric nursing homes enjoy the same status as wards in rest and nursing homes. Of the 20 000 existing and occupied beds in the psychiatric hospital sector, nearly 5 000 will be converted to nursing home status. Payments by patients in these psychiatric nursing homes will be considerably higher than in the hospital sector since the patient must bear the total cost of board and lodging;
- A higher payment will be required from patients who have resided more than five years in psychiatric hospitals;
- An increase in the quality of care in acute wards in psychiatric hospitals: the personnel will be increased from ten medical staff per 30 beds to 12 or even 14 in hospitals with an average stay of less than one year;
- A programme to create sheltered housing, away from the hospital environment, with an anticipated ratio of one member of medical staff per eight places: it is estimated that nearly 3 000 places in sheltered housing will be created.
- A co-ordination scheme between the various ambulatory and institutional psychiatric services: the scheme will be voluntary but a budget has been set aside for its administration.

GROWTH AND PERFORMANCE

According to OECD figures, Belgian health expenditure, converted at purchasing power parity exchange rates, was $879 per capita in 1987, 16 % above that in the United Kingdom, 80 % of that in France and 43 % of that in the United States. This was almost exactly the level which would be expected on the basis of a regression line linking health expenditure per capita with GDP per capita (Schieber and Poullier, 1989).

However, alternative estimates (Wouters, Spinnewyn and Pacolet, 1988) which have compared Belgian health expenditure with Dutch health expenditure, using the same method of estimation as that of the Netherlands Ministry of Health, suggest that Belgian health expenditure is actually 10 % above the level reported to the OECD. This would put Belgium above the regression line which links per capita health expenditure with per capita GDP, and 30 % above the United Kingdom, which has a similar standard of living.

The difficulties with the measurement of health expenditure extend to comparisons over time. Again, according to OECD figures, real health expenditure rose briskly by 21 % between 1980 and 1990. The share of health expenditure in GDP rose from 6.6 % in 1980 to 7.6 % in 1990. This was the fastest proportionate increase over this period among the seven countries in this study, although it was much slower than the apparent rate of increase in Belgium between 1970 and 1980. These comparisons must be treated with caution, however, because it is believed that the scope of the expenditure figures estimated for Belgium has changed slightly over time.

However, the government has succeeded in its policies of limiting the size and improving the efficiency of the acute hospital sector. The number of beds in general hospitals fell from 7.04 per head of population in 1983 to 6.29 per head of population in 1988. Despite this reduction in capacity, average length of stay fell by over 10 % and admission rates rose slightly over the same period (Ministère de la Santé publique, 1988).

For several other sectors, however, the system found itself in a vicious circle. The rising volume of services, induced by fee-for-service incentives, was met by real cuts in the level of fees, only for the effect to be nullified by a further rise in volume. This was because providers strove to maintain or increase their real incomes. This was particularly true for laboratory services until the payment system was reformed at the end of the decade (Kesenne and Cannoodt, 1989).

According to OECD (1987), Schieber, Poullier and Greenwald (1991) and the figures in Table 10.2 in Chapter 10, Belgium has fairly typical rates of: total in-patient beds per 1 000 population; hospital admissions per 1 000; and average length of stay in hospitals. However, it has exceptionally high numbers of physicians per 1 000 (close to those observed for Spain); above-average physician contacts per capita and an exceptionally low ratio of physicians' average income to average employee income. Young GPs often have to rely on their wife's earnings to supplement their incomes. There are no reports of significant hospital waiting lists. As Table 10.3 shows, perinatal mortality is fairly representative of the levels found in the other countries in this study, and it decreased at a fairly typical rate between 1980 and 1986.

CONTINUING DEBATE

Two issues continue to dominate the debate on health policy within Belgium: how to control the cost of health care within the context of health insurance and who will pay for the higher cost of health care.

As part of the debate, the Minister for Social Affairs organised a ''round table'' conference in 1989. One of the main issues discussed by the participants was establishing the relevant responsibilities of all the partners in the health care sector. The conference discussed financial responsibility as well as the role of arrangements and agreements on fees, medical supervision and the administrative control in health insurance.

In its final report, the conference's finance working group brought forward a set of principles related to the financing of health care:

- Mixed contributory and tax financing has to be maintained, thus justifying the role and functions of all parties involved in the management of social security;
- Social security contributions should not increase and the health insurance share should not rise at the expense of other branches of social security;
- General taxation should cover the bulk of health expenditure, apart from contributions, but it should not constitute a fixed percentage of the total and it is unlikely that, in future, it could be increased substantially;
- There is little scope for increasing cost-sharing by patients.

The conference's final report considered the control of expenditure, but offered nothing more than a general approach to budget allocation. The report recommended that an overall, central government allocation should be distributed to the various sectors under the supervision of committees. However, nowhere did the report make clear how the committees should act. The report also recommended that methods of global budgeting should be developed and applied.

Following these proposals, the government introduced a cost-containment bill in December 1990, which modifies the law on health insurance and provides for:

- The fixing of a global budget for health care expenditures and several separate budgets for each sector;
- The obligation to implement correction mechanisms when the global or partial budgets are exceeded;
- The creation of a budget control commission entrusted with the supervision of the achievement of budgetary targets and with the task of proposing adjustments to them;
- Powers for the Minister to intervene when the care providers and the *mutualités* do not succeed in meeting their budgetary targets.

The bill has important implications for the balance between government regulation and self-regulation of the health care system. Rather than granting more financial responsibility to the *mutualités,* it strengthens the role of government in controlling the level of health expenditure.

It seems that a clearer division of labour may emerge in the regulation of the Belgian health care system. The government may assume full responsibility for macro-economic efficiency – or the overall control of health expenditure – and leave the patients, insurers and providers to pursue micro-economic efficiency within a firm framework of solidarity and global budgets. In some respects, this may allow the government to step back from detailed intervention. Since consumers will not be cost-conscious, the *mutualités* will be responsible for bargaining with the providers about fees and charges, and to share the burden of cost-containment with the government. Likewise, since consumers are usually in a weak position to judge the technical quality of care, it will be the responsibility of the providers and the *mutualités* to develop better quality assurance procedures.

However, it seems likely that Belgium can continue to rely on its strong traditions of consumer choice and autonomy of provider to ensure competition among providers, a high level of responsiveness to demands and a high level of patient satisfaction. Indeed, a firmer grip on macro-economic efficiency may be the best way, in the long term, to preserve *la médecine libérale* and the benefits which it can bring in terms of patient choice and provider autonomy.

Notes

1. This chapter is based on a paper by: J. Hermesse, J. Kesenne and L. Moorthamer, *Alliance Nationale des Mutualités Chrétiennes;* and A. de Wever and J. Beeckmans, *Ministère des Affaires Sociales,* Belgium.
2. These figures are estimates for the sole year 1987. They are slightly higher than the OECD Secretariat's estimates because they include expenditures by provinces and local communities, but also some headings that appear to be classified under environment, hygiene and amenities in other countries' accounts.

References

Blanplain, J. E. (1984), "The health services system in Belgium", in *Reorienting Health Services,* edited by C. O. Pannenborg, A. van der Werff, G. B. Hirsch, and K. Barnard, NATO Conference Series, Plenum Press, New York.

Courrier Hebdomadaire (1989), CRISP, No. 1255-1256.

De Cooman, E. and Marchand, M. (1987), "Rules and Incentives for Hospitals: the Belgian Financing System", *Health Policy,* 7.

Feltesse, P. (1988), *Aperçu de la situation des hôpitaux dans les pays de la CEE,* ANMC (note interne).

Grinberg, G. and Dekeyser, T., *Assurance-maladie: Financement et régulation.*

Groot, L. M. J., van Daele, D. and Cannoodt, L. (1986), *Evaluation of hospital programmation. Part I: Acute hospital care.* December (in Dutch).

Heesters, J. and Kesenne, J. (1985), "The financing of health care in Belgium and the Netherlands". LCM Dossier, November 3 (in Dutch).

Hermesse, J. (1986), "Hospital Financing in Belgium: Recent Changes and Future Options", *Health Policy,* 6.

Huybrechs, J. (1990), *The sickness insurance system in Belgium: structure, problems, perspectives 1992,* LCM Dossier, March (in Dutch and German).

INAMI, Service des Soins de Santé, Comité de Gestion, Note C.S. No. 90/126.

Kesenne, J. (1989), "The 'Round Table' on the Sickness Insurance. The financial problems", *De Gids op Maatschappelijk Gebied,* 80.5 (in Dutch).

Kesenne, J. (1989), "The financing of Clinical Biology", *M-informatie,* 139, October (in Dutch).

Kesenne, J. and Cannoodt, L. (1989), "Laboratory Testing in the Belgian Health Care System", typescript.

Ministère de la Santé publique (1988), *Annuaire Statistique des Etablissements de Soins,* January.

Nonneman, W. L. M. (1990), "Health Care in Belgium", *Competitive Health Care in Europe: Future Prospects,* edited by Casparie, A. F., Hermans, H. E. G. M. and Paelinck, J. H. P., Dartmouth Publishing Co. Ltd.

Nys, H. and Quaethoven, P. (1984), "Health Services in Belgium", *Comparative Health Systems,* edited by Raffel M. W., Pennsylvania State University Press.

OECD (1987), *Financing and Delivering Health Care,* OCDE, Paris.

Poullier, J. P. and Sandier, S. (1988), "Les dépenses de santé dans la CEE", *Prospective et Santé,* No. 47-48, pp. 17-24.

Schieber, G. and J., Poullier, J. P. (1989), "International Health Care Expenditure Trends", *Health Affairs,* Fall, pp. 169-177.

Schieber, G. J., Poullier, J. P. and Greenwald, L. M. (1991), ''Health Care Systems in Twenty-Four Countries'', *Health Affairs,* Fall.

van den Heuvel, R. and Sacrez, A. (1982), ''Cost-Containment in Health Insurance: the case of Belgium'', in *The Public-Private Mix for Health,* edited by McLachlan G. and Maynard A., Nuffield Provincial Hospitals Trust, London.

Wouters, R., Spinnewyn, H. and Pacolet, J. (1988), *Het Profijt van de Non-Profijt,* Koning Boudewijnstichting en het Hoger Instituut voor de Arbeid, Brussel (in Dutch).

Schieber, G.J., Poullier, J.-P. and Greenwald, L.M. (1991), "Health Care Systems in Twenty-Four Countries", *Health*

Van den Heuvel, W.J. van (1980), "Health Commitment in Health Insurance in ...

... (1983), *Medical Care*, ...

Vaughan, R., ...

Chapter 4

THE REFORM OF THE HEALTH SYSTEM IN FRANCE

INTRODUCTION

The French health care system is arguably the most complex of those examined in this report. It combines universal rational health insurance, involving significant cost-sharing and supplementary insurance on the financing side with a pluralist system of provision, involving both independent and public providers, on the supply side. There is a considerable diversity of methods by which providers receive payment. The first part of this chapter describes the main features of this health care system which, in many ways, owes more to the accumulation of layers of history than to the exercise of common design principles at one point in time.

Several French commentators have drawn attention to a tension which exists between, on the one hand, the socialist principles which are embodied in national, health insurance and, on the other, the liberal principles implied by independent medical practice (*la médecine libérale*). The enforced and uneasy "marriage" between the two principles has been described as "a costly union" (Rodwin, 1981*a*) because both contain incentives to expand medical care. Although there have been no structural changes in recent years to the social insurance system, the government has introduced a number of modest reforms aimed at stabilizing overall spending and improving performance. The second part of the chapter describes these reforms, and goes on to consider some evidence on how the system has responded over the past decade.

Persistent difficulties with the funding and operation of the health care system have generated a debate within France about the need for more fundamental, structural reforms. The chapter ends by describing and evaluating some of the options which have been considered.

HEALTH CARE SYSTEM DESCRIBED

In terms of the models set out in Chapter 2, the French health care system is a complicated blend of at least four different sub-systems. The basis is a public reimbursement model. This is blended with a public contract model in the case of ambulatory care and private hospitals, and overlaid by a public integrated model in the case of public hospitals. The resulting public system is supplemented by voluntary insurance according to the reimbursement model.

Chart 4.1 shows some of the main features of the organisation and financing of medical care in the late 1980s. At the bottom left of the diagram is the population, 60 % of whom are reckoned to become patients or demand health services in any one year. At the bottom right are the providers of health services. At the top are the third-party payers, both public and private. Service flows are shown as solid lines and financial flows as broken lines.

The providers have been separated into: public health services; pharmacists; independent general practitioners and specialists; municipal medical centres with salaried doctors; public hospitals with salaried doctors (accounting for about two-thirds of beds); and private hospitals, profit-making and non-profit-making, usually with fee-for-service doctors (accounting for the remaining one-third of beds). In addition (not shown in the diagram) there are various long-term care homes, residential nursing facilities and home help services financed variously by: the health insurance system; the old-age branch of social security; the social assistance scheme; and by private means.

The third-party payers have been separated into: the statutory health insurance funds or *Caisses Nationales* (quasi autonomous, non-governmental bodies charged with operating the compulsory national health insurance scheme which covers 99 % of the population); *mutuelles* or friendly societies (non-profit insurers) and private insurers which provide essentially supplementary voluntary insurance for about 80 % of the population; and public bodies, such as the Ministry of Health, which fund mainly public health services and provide some capital

Chart 4.1 Detail of relationships in the French health care system in 1988

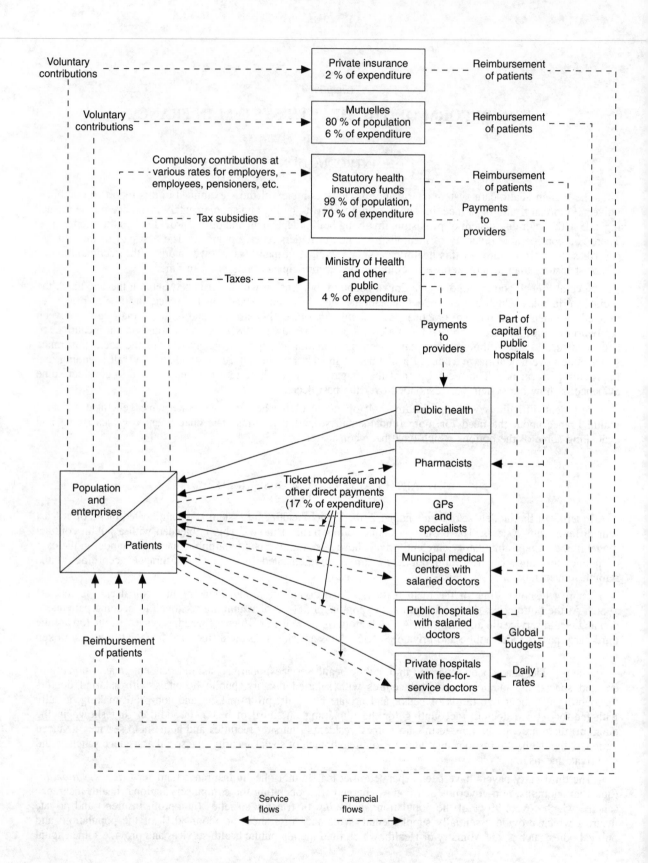

for public providers. The insurers offer benefits in the form of reimbursement of patients for most ambulatory care and direct payments to providers for most hospital care, subject to cost-sharing in both cases.

Social insurance accounts for over 70 % of total health care expenditure, the *mutuelles* for about 6 %, the public sector for about 4 %, private insurers for about 2 %, leaving about 17 % for out-of-pocket payments by households (CREDES, 1989).

RELATIONSHIP BETWEEN PATIENTS AND PROVIDERS

The relationship between patient and doctor is still governed largely by the principles of *la médecine libérale* which were laid down in the 1920s:
- Free choice of doctor by the patient;
- Freedom of prescription and location by the doctor;
- Fee-for-service payment by the patient, ideally agreed between the two parties without interference; and
- Confidentiality.

The only deviation from these principles is the fact that the government introduced a national fee schedule (or *nomenclature*) for independent doctors in 1960, and employs about one-third of doctors full-time on salaries and another one-third part-time on salaries, mainly in public hospitals.

Thus, the patient who seeks primary medical care can choose to consult any medical practitioner. There is no gatekeeper role for the GP. The patient pays for the service directly and the fee will reflect the precise service and whether the doctor is permitted to extra bill. Similarly, if a prescription is required, the patient usually goes to a private pharmacist to have it dispensed and makes a direct payment for the drugs. The patient can later claim back a proportion of the bills paid from the social security, subject to a cost-sharing arrangement which excludes from reimbursement a percentage of the standard cost (the *ticket modérateur*) and any extra billing. Direct billing of the sickness fund by the pharmacists with patients paying only the *ticket modérateur* is, however, gaining currency.

Consultations with a doctor are normally subject to a *ticket modérateur* of 25 % of the conventional fee; the rate for "necessary" drugs is 30 % but "comfort" drugs attract 60 %. About 10 % of the insured are exempt from the *ticket modérateur* because they are suffering from long-term illnesses. If the patient has supplementary voluntary insurance, a further proportion of the bill can be claimed back, normally the full *ticket modérateur;* extra billing may be wholly or partly refunded depending on the insurance cover provided.

There are also over 2 000 municipal health centres where salaried doctors provide ambulatory and preventive care. These play an important role in providing services for the poor because the patient is only required to pay the proportion of the bill which is not covered by social security. In some cases, this co-payment is waived.

If hospital care is required, the patient, again, has freedom of choice between public and private hospitals, both of which are covered without discrimination under national health insurance. Money follows the patient in the case of private hospitals, but public hospitals are subject to global budgets. About two-thirds of beds are in public hospitals with salaried full-time or part-time doctors. About one-third are in private, mainly for-profit hospitals with fee-for-service doctors. These are often owned by doctors. Public hospitals tend to be large, well equipped and under a duty to deal with accident and emergencies. They have a limited dispensation to treat private patients. Private hospitals tend to be smaller and to specialise in elective surgery, obstetrics, or long-term care. The relationship between the two has been partly complementary but is becoming increasingly competitive as some private clinics acquire the equipment to tackle more complicated cases.

In principle, most patients are required to pay for public hospital care and to seek reimbursement, but, in practice, the *caisses* meet the bills leaving the patient responsible only for nominal co-payments (at the end of 1991, FF 55.00 per day for in-patients with an additional co-insurance of 20 % for short-term stays up to 30 days, if the patient is not exempt). Only 4 % of hospital expenditure is financed directly by patients.

There is an extensive network of long-term care institutions which cater for about 4 % of the population over 60 years of age. There is also domiciliary support in the form of home nursing and home help services (Rozenkier, 1990).

Almost the entire population is covered by the statutory health insurance scheme which is part of the social security system. The scheme accounts for over 70 % of total medical care expenditure. The basis for the membership of a fund is occupational. There is one large fund for salaried workers – *Caisse Nationale d'Assurance Maladie des Travailleurs Salariés* (CNAMTS) – which accounts for nearly 80 % of the compulsorily insured, including pensioners and dependants. About 15 smaller funds cover, for example, farmers and agricultural workers, the self-employed and special groups of employees, such as miners and transport workers. A safety net of medical assistance exists for those who have never had a stable occupation and who cannot afford cost-sharing (about 2.8 million people).

Contributions vary between the schemes but all are income-related. For the CNAMTS, the employer's and employee's contributions were, respectively, 12.6 % and 6.8 % of the total salary in July 1992 without an upper earnings limit. Given a further contribution of perhaps 2.5 % of salary to a *mutuelle* or private insurer, this means that French workers are paying over a fifth of their earnings (including the employer's contribution) for health insurance. In addition, employers pay for a separate, work accident scheme. The self-employed are liable for the whole contribution on their declared income. Since 1980, most pensioners have paid a sum equivalent to 1 % of their pension. There are various cross subsidies between the schemes because of imbalances between contributions and benefits. The State also provides the system with a small tax subsidy, partly funded by a levy on car insurance and by alcohol and tobacco excise taxes.

The schemes provide both cash benefits (sick pay) and benefits in kind (for ambulatory care, drugs, maternity care, dental care, medical goods and hospitalisation). Cash benefits are excluded from the expenditure figures quoted below. Most of the benefits in kind for ambulatory care are provided in the form of partial reimbursement of medical bills. However, there is considerable direct payment for hospital care by the various funds.

The CNAMTS and other statutory health insurers are quasi autonomous, non-governmental bodies with national headquarters and regional and local networks. They are subject to national and local management by employers associations and trade unions. However, they are also closely regulated by central government in their carrying out of what is essentially a public function. In particular, contribution rates, the fee schedules negotiated with providers and pharmaceutical prices are under the control of central government.

The *mutuelles* (of which there are several thousands with small memberships) and the private insurers play only a supplementary role in the system. They cover the *ticket modérateur,* some extra billing, and a few benefits not covered by the social security scheme. The *mutuelles* are usually organised for groups of employees or professions, and contributions are based on the solidarity principle. Private insurers offer their services on the open market and levy flat-rate premiums according to actuarial risk and benefits.

RELATIONSHIP BETWEEN THIRD-PARTY PAYERS AND PROVIDERS

In the ambulatory care and private hospital sector (the "liberal" sector), relationships between the statutory insurance bodies and the doctors have been characterised by a long struggle between the desire for cost-containment on the part of the insurers and the desire to preserve *la médecine libérale* on the part of most doctors (Godt, 1985).

Since 1960, the law has provided for a national fee schedule for GPs and specialists to be negotiated between the insurers and the doctors' representatives. The fee schedule or *nomenclature* consists of three parts: a list of over 4 000 procedures grouped under about 50 alpha-numeric codes (or "key letters"); a relative value-scale for each procedure; and a set of monetary multipliers for the alpha-numeric codes. The doctor bills for the number of points under each alpha-numeric code. The list and the relative values are changed infrequently and the latter generally fail to reflect the relative costs of different procedures. The monetary multipliers are generally re-negotiated annually. The alpha-numeric codes exist to preserve patient confidentiality: consultations are undifferentiated, for example. This also serves to conceal from the insurers much of the detailed composition of each doctor's workload.

Individual doctors are free to choose not to contract with the social security system; in the late 1980s about 97 % did so (they are *conventionnés*). However, contracted doctors have been free to choose to practise within one of two sectors.

- In *sector 1* doctors agree to abide by the negotiated fee schedule in exchange for a free pension package and personal health insurance. This, in turn, guarantees the patient reimbursement at 75 % of the fee schedule.
- In *sector 2* doctors are free to set their own fees (with "tact and moderation") but must pay their own pension and insurance contributions. This, in turn, exposes the patient to extra billing (*les dépassements*) because patient reimbursement by the social security funds is based on the fixed-fee schedule.

As many as 26 % of doctors had opted to practise in sector 2 in 1990 – mainly specialists and doctors who worked in large cities. This was partly a result of the fact that the fee schedule made no adjustments either for the prestige of the doctor or geographical cost variations. As a result, it became difficult to find sector 1 specialists in the centre of cities such as Paris and Lyons.

The statutory insurers have little or no control over the volume of medical services or the location of doctors. However, they do monitor the volume of each doctor's activity and feed back the results in the hope that this will influence his or her volume of activity. Excessive prescribing may be sanctioned.

France operates a positive list for drugs. Pharmaceuticals have to be approved for reimbursement at a price set, product by product, by the French Medicines Directorate. Innovative products are allowed higher prices as a contribution to research and development costs but, if a drug offers no therapeutic advantages over its rivals, it is only admitted to the list if its price is below theirs. Since 1990, pharmacists have been paid according to a sliding scale which is related to the cost of the drug dispensed. Generally, the patient pays the pharmacist directly for the drugs and the patient is later reimbursed by the social security fund. There is, however, some direct payment of pharmacists by the *caisses* for patients who are exempt from charges.

Public hospitals and some private non-profit hospitals have had global, prospective budgets for operating expenses since 1984 or 1985. These are shared between the relevant local statutory insurers in proportion to the number of bed days consumed in their catchment area. Doctors in public hospitals are salaried. The budgets include depreciation and interest on capital and are based on historical levels of expenditure. A rate of increase for all global budgets is set centrally, with little scope for local deviation. The budgets are made available in monthly instalments. It is government policy to move towards standardization of the level of budget across all hospitals according to workload.

Investment expenditure in public hospitals comes mainly from self-financing (principally from depreciation receipts) and from loans. Government grants, mainly for large, new schemes, account for only about 10 % of total new investment. These methods of funding tend to favour hospitals which are already well endowed.

Most private hospitals are reimbursed on a per diem basis for in-patient care, with separate fee-for-service payments for physician services under the same convention, which applies to ambulatory care. The rates cover depreciation and interest on capital. They are negotiated between the hospitals and the statutory insurers under government guidelines about the permitted annual rate of growth of prices. From 1992, a form of capping has been established, which however excludes day surgery.

The statutory health insurance system plays an important part in financing long-term care, much of which is provided by the hospital system. There is also support for home nursing and for medical care in nursing and residential homes for the elderly. Other sources of third-party finance include the old-age branch of the general social security scheme and social assistance (Rozenkier, 1990).

GOVERNMENT PLANNING AND REGULATION

The health care system is closely supervised by the government with relatively little reliance on self-regulation. Rather than allowing the social security *caisses* to exercise a countervailing power, government takes the lead in controlling costs and in planning. It seems that the *caisses* answer to employers and employees and, as a result, are subject to local pressures in their negotiations with doctors and private hospitals. In many ways, they act more like passive funders than active buyers. At times, they even form temporary alliances with the independent providers against the government.

The main ways in which the government exercises control over the system include:

- Regulation of social security contribution rates: the implicit policy appears to be that the growth of health expenditure should remain in step with the growth of GDP;
- Control of the global budgets for public hospitals;
- Control of wages and posts in public hospitals;

Table 4.1. **Government price and volume regulation**[1]

	Control of Price		Control of Volume	
	Rate of Increase	Price per Unit	Activity	Investment
Public hospitals	Global budgets and wage controls			Beds, major equipment
Private hospitals	Per diem[2]	x	x	Beds, major equipment
Independent doctors	*Nomenclature* and key letters		x	Number of medical students
Independent non-medical providers (laboratories, ambulances, nursing care)	*Nomenclature* and key letters[3]			
Pharmaceuticals	Public reimbursement price		x	Number of pharmacies

1. This table was suggested by Christine Meyer, *Commissariat Général du Plan*.
2. With some capping from 1992 (except for day surgery).
3. With some capping from 1992.

- Supervision of the negotiation of fees and prices for doctors and private hospitals and direct control of the prices paid by the statutory insurers for drugs and medical goods (from 1992, part of the negotiation process may be transferred to the *caisses*);
- Planning for the acquisition of equipment and new construction by both public and private hospitals (via a *carte sanitaire*);
- Control of the numbers of students entering the second year of medical school so as to constrain the increase in the number of doctors.
- A (high) ceiling on the number of pharmacies per capita.

As Table 4.1 shows, the main central government controls operate on prices and on new investment. Activity is largely uncontrolled, apart from the indirect effect of global budgets on public hospitals.

RECENT REFORMS

The most important reform of the past decade was the introduction of global, prospective budgeting for public hospitals (in 1984 for larger hospitals and 1985 for the remainder). With the aim of containing costs, global budgeting replaced a system of controlled rates of increase of per diem prices, which itself replaced a system of more or less retrospective cost-based pricing. The per diem prices gave incentives to hospital managers to maximise average length of stay. Global budgeting provides much tighter overall cost control combined with increased management freedom at the local level. Since the early 1980s, tighter budgeting in public hospitals has been aided by wage controls.

Another reform which had important consequences was the introduction, in the 1980s, of freedom of access for ambulatory care doctors to a sector 2 within the convention governing medical fees. This allowed doctors to opt for extra billing. The agreement was combined with a provision for the patients of such doctors to be reimbursed no more than a fixed percentage of the nationally negotiated fee. This replaced earlier arrangements under which the privilege of free price-fixing was given only to a small number of physicians, chosen for their scientific reputation, and patients were reimbursed at a fixed percentage of the actual fee charged. The aim seems to have been to shift some of the burden of financing rising medical fees to the patient (or his/her complementary insurance). The doctors' new freedom to join sector 2 was, presumably, to be tempered by the full exposure of patients to the cost of extra billing.

However, the drift of doctors into sector 2 caused problems of access to specialists for patients on lower incomes in large cities. As Enthoven (1988) points out, when the supply curve is inelastic, the freedom of providers to extra bill allows medical fees to rise towards the sum of the insurance payments plus the pre-insurance fees, and consumers will, in effect, be uninsured. Furthermore, the growing rewards for doctors in sector 1 began to threaten the government's position in bargaining over fees in both sectors. In 1989, the government decided to freeze further access to sector 2. After protracted negotiations between the insurers, the government and the medical unions, and strikes by junior hospital doctors whose careers might have been blighted by such a freeze, a new agreement was reached in March 1990. This allowed for:

- A temporary freeze on access to sector 2 except for a specified sub-group of junior hospital doctors;
- A requirement for doctors already in sector 2 to devote 25 % of their practice to services provided in exchange for the nationally negotiated fees, or to free care or to other public service;
- Payments for continuing medical education by doctors financed by a small levy on fees;
- An immediate five-franc increase in fees.

The government has also introduced a number of minor reforms or "plans" during the 1980s and early 1990s, mostly in an attempt to stem the rise of costs. They included:

- The removal of the upper earnings limit for employees' contributions in 1980 and for employers' contributions in 1984;
- Periodic minor increases in cost-sharing for drugs and the introduction of the nominal charge for hospital care;
- The introduction of a negative list of drugs, not reimbursable by the statutory insurers, in 1983;
- Reforms of medical education, including a tightening of controls on medical students which reduced the numbers graduating from 6 400 in 1980 to 4 100 in 1988;
- Basing the remuneration of pharmacists on a sliding scale in relation to the price of drugs instead of on a fixed proportion of the price;
- The creation, in 1989, of a national agency for health technology assessment;
- Measures to encourage preventive health care in certain regions;
- Further measures to restrict reimbursement of pharmaceuticals in 1986, 1990 and 1991;
- The limitation of laboratory and surgical theatre costs in private hospitals by including the former in the per diem payment from 1991 and capping the latter at the 1990 level. A medicalised information system is due to be created from 1993 to link payments to real throughputs;
- The negotiation of agreements for pathology laboratory services and ambulance services putting a ceiling on outlays (at the 1990 level) in 1991;
- Negotiation in 1991-1992 of similar agreements with private practice nurses and other health professions, only the agreement with self-employed physicians failing to be ratified by the contracting parties.

GROWTH AND PERFORMANCE

To summarise: the French health care system combines universal, national health insurance with a pluralist system of provision and fee-for-service payment for a large part of medical care. The government has exercised strong controls over fees and prices, but only weak controls over the volume of inputs and activity. The system can be characterised as mainly "demand-led", at least until the introduction of global budgeting for public hospitals in 1984/1985.

It is not surprising, perhaps, that according to OECD figures the share of health expenditure in GDP grew rapidly between 1960 and 1985 – from 4.2 % in 1960, to 5.8 % in 1970, to 7.6 % in 1980, to 8.5 in 1985, and to 8.8 % in 1990. France shared with Belgium a considerably faster rate of growth of the health expenditure share of GDP in the 1980s than in the other five countries in the study. This doubling of the share in 25 years paralleled closely experience in the United States, albeit at lower shares in France at the beginning and end of the period (Schieber and Poullier, 1989). However, whereas health expenditure growth was accelerating in the United States between 1970 and 1990, it was decelerating in France. Moreover, measured relative health care prices fell steadily over this period in France whereas they rose on average in the United States between 1975 and 1980 and between 1980 and 1990 (Sandier, 1989b; OECD, forthcoming).

Health expenditure per head of population in 1987 was US$ 1 105 at purchasing power parity, close to that of the Netherlands and Germany, half that of the United States and nearly 50 % more than that of the United Kingdom. Actual health expenditure per capita was slightly above that which would be expected on the basis of a regression line linking GDP to health expenditure in major OECD countries (Schieber and Poullier, 1989).

Again, according to OECD statistics, updated by Table 10.2 in Chapter 10, France has above-average levels of consultations with doctors, medicines prescribed outside hospitals, acute hospital beds, and acute hospital admissions. However, average length of stay in acute hospitals is well below that of Germany and the Netherlands. France also has a relatively high level of doctors per 1 000 population (2.6 in 1989). The number of doctors per 1 000 doubled between 1971 and 1987 and this coincided with a fall in GPs' average earnings from over three times the national average wage to a little over twice the national average wage (Sandier, 1989a). The volume of services per doctor also rose steadily.

What impact, if any, did these trends have on the health status of the French population? It is difficult to be confident about answering this question, partly because health care is not the only factor which determines health. However, OECD figures (Schieber *et al.,* 1991) suggest that, in 1989, France was a middling country in terms of expectation of life at birth (72.7 years for males, OECD average 72.2; and 80.1 years for females, OECD average 79.0).

France also appears to have had favourable trends in "avoidable" mortality – deaths from selected causes which doctors believe to be amenable to medical interventions (perinatal mortality, tuberculosis, and stroke in the age group 35-64). According to Charlton and Velez (1986), "avoidable" mortality rates fell more rapidly in France between 1956 and 1978 than in England and Wales, the United States, Italy and Sweden, although deaths from such causes fell even more steeply in Japan. The World Health Organisaion data on potential years of life lost between 1960 and 1989 reinforce this observation (OECD, forthcoming).

Some of the reforms introduced during the 1980s have had a visible, if temporary, effect on national statistics. The share of GDP devoted to health expenditure was stabilized between 1985 and 1987 at 8.5 % and has been increasing more moderately through 1990. This was due mainly to the global budget for public hospitals. Hospital expenditure fell as a proportion of total health expenditure from 47 % in 1985 to about 44 % in 1990. This was not achieved without provoking strikes among public hospital workers and complaints about unfair competition from private hospitals (CREDES, 1989).

The government was less successfull in containing the costs of ambulatory care. Expenditure per capita rose by more than 50 % between 1985 and 1990, mainly because of extra billing and rising volume. There was an increase in the number of doctors permitted to extra bill (those of sector 2) from 7 % of all doctors in 1980 to 26 % in 1989. This, together with raised co-payments, caused out-of-pocket payments to rise from 15.6 % of health expenditure in 1980 to 19.9 % in 1988 (using a slightly narrower definition of health expenditure than for the figures at the beginning of the chapter). This is threatening to perpetuate a slight tendency for consumption of medical care to be positively associated with high level of income and social class (CREDES, 1989).

Increased cost-sharing, however, has had little effect in restraining the growth of health expenditure. Volume continues to rise rapidly, despite the feedback of data on the activities of physicians in independent practice. Overall, the growth of health expenditure accelerated after 1987 and the share of GDP devoted to health care rose from 8.5 to 8.8 % in 1990. Faced with a deficit in the social security system, the government was obliged to raise the employee contribution rate from July 1991.

STRENTGHS, WEAKNESSES AND POTENTIAL SOLUTIONS

France has enjoyed considerable success in meeting the policy objectives for health care set out in Chapter 1. The health care system has provided high standards of services to the whole population, achieving considerable equity in access. It has protected the incomes of consumers when they are sick. Compared with past decades, the growth of health expenditure has been slowed in the 1990s. There is a considerable freedom of choice for consumers and a corresponding high level of autonomy for providers. This means that there is much consumer-led competition in the system and micro-economic efficiency has been achieved in the sense that ambulatory care doctors and private hospitals are responsive to patients and consumer satisfaction is high (Blendon *et al,* 1990).

However, certain persistent difficulties remain, including: a relatively rapid rate of growth of health expenditure contributing to recurrent deficits on the social security budget; rapid increases in the volume of some acute services, leading to probable waste and unnecessary care; deficiencies in long-term care; and concerns about the efficiency of public hospitals. To some extent, these difficulties arise from circumstances outside the control of the government, such as the ageing of the population and the continued development of expensive medical techniques. However, they are also the result of inappropriate incentives for patients and providers; and management systems which are far from ideal.

So far as patients themselves are concerned, near universal health insurance means that they have little disincentive to restrain their initial demand for care. Although France has high cost-sharing under social insurance for ambulatory care, the effects are generally undermined by the widespread use of supplementary insurance. In any event, patients are not usually well enough informed to question the treatment and prescribing decisions of their doctors. Meanwhile, the growth of extra billing under sector 2 has contributed to inequity as much as to cost-consciousness among patients.

Turning to doctors in ambulatory care and in private hospitals, fee-for-service reimbursement and the growth in the number of doctors have provided powerful incentives for growth in the volume of certain types of care – for example, prescribing and diagnostic tests. It seems likely that doctors pursue a target income. So, while the government has been successful in controlling the level of scheduled fees, the effect has been undermined by the growth in the volume of services per doctor. In the case of pharmaceuticals, the combination of one of the highest prescribing rates in the OECD with one of the lowest levels of pharmaceutical prices has not served to encourage the pursuit of research and development by the French pharmaceutical industry. The government is investigating alternative methods of controlling pharmaceutical prices, starting with the proposal to create a medicines agency in 1992 empowered to assume several regulatory functions hitherto dispersed in several bureaus.

In other areas, such as prevention, public hospitals and long-term care, the growth of services has been rationed. In the case of long-term care, the supply of care is not keeping up with the growing needs caused by an ageing population. The result is that unacceptable financial burdens are sometimes falling on the elderly or their families. There is not always a clear relationship between the design of the incentive mechanisms, the shifting needs of the population and the broader goals of health policy.

Global budgets and wage limits have given central government firmer control over the rate of growth of expenditure in public hospitals. However, the tensions generated by imposing tight budgetary restraints on public hospitals have been exacerbated by being run alongside an apparently less restrictive system for most private hospitals. Moreover, it is not easy with global budgets to provide rewards for treating more patients or for raising productivity. Money no longer follows the patient into public hospitals. The possibility that surpluses may be claimed back reduces the incentive to lower costs. It could be argued that there is too much autonomy and stimulation for private hospitals and not enough of either for public hospitals. The former are currently subject to negotiated ceilings, as indicated below.

Several aspects of the system discourage self-regulation or make it ineffective. In particular, central government tends to be drawn into periodic attempts to stem the rise in costs. The successive minor reforms or "plans" have had favourable effects in the short term but have failed to prevent the reappearance of deficits in the social security system after a year or two.

It is possible that, with the steady accumulation of some relatively modest and short-term reforms, the distinctive French mixture of national health insurance, public hospitals and *la médecine libérale* can be adapted to achieve the government's policy aims for health. Towards such an end, a Hospital Reform Law was adopted by Parliament in the spring of 1991. The main points, which are designed to create a more level playing field between public and private hospitals, include:

- Putting hospital planning on a regional basis;
- Giving more autonomy to public hospitals in setting their investment budgets and in creating and suppressing posts;
- Extending the *carte sanitaire* to the *use* of expensive medical techniques rather than only to the acquisition of equipment;
- Requiring evaluation of activity by and accreditation of private hospitals;
- Requiring private hospitals to enter into agreements (*conventions*) with the *caisses* specifying their expected volume of service.

The government has also examined proposals to experiment with moving away from product-by-product regulation of pharmaceutical prices to a form of global budgeting of pharmaceutical companies, rather like the Pharmaceutical Price Regulation Scheme in the United Kingdom. Lack of consensus within the industry as well as among decision-makers failed to convert the study process into actual experiments.

It may well be the case, however, that the government's policy aims cannot be achieved without more fundamental, structural reforms. Here, there are several options which the government might consider. One possibility would be to follow the Belgian and German directions: to impose global budgets for the services offered by the independent providers, as well as for the services offered by the public hospitals, while, at the same time, encouraging a more active buying role by the *caisses*. This might allow the government to step back somewhat and might improve the climate for discussions about new methods of paying providers for some services. Mixed payment systems, involving elements of fee for service, capitation and salary, might break the vicious circles involving ever lower fees and ever higher volumes.

Alternatively, the government might follow the Dutch example by encouraging the creation of managed markets, both for health insurance and for health services themselves. In this connection, Giraud and Launois (1985), and Launois *et al.* (1985) have proposed a model for managed competition based on Enthoven's "consumer choice health plan" (Enthoven, 1980). This would involve a set of institutions new to France – *réseaux de soins coordonnés* (RSCs) – based on the "health management organisation" (HMO) concept in the United States. Since HMOs combine both insurance and provision, the proposals envisage consumer choice over both.

The proposed model would involve six principles:

a) The retention of compulsory, income-related contributions to national health insurance; that is to say, the retention of "solidarity";

b) The creation of a network of insurers/suppliers, the *réseaux de soins coordonnés* (RSCs) building on the existing actors in the health care system;

c) The promotion of care of the whole person (including prevention) by RSCs;

d) The funding of RSCs mainly by annually transferable risk-related capitation payments made available through the statutory insurance system;

e) Cost-sharing by consumers not when they require care, but in the cost of the risk-adjusted capitation payments, roughly equal, on average, to the proportion represented by the current *tickets modérateurs* (20 %);

f) The promotion of competition between RSCs, between RSCs and fee-for-service providers, and between providers competing for the business of RSCs.

The aim of such a system would be for consumer choice of insurer, based on awareness of costs and quality, to engender competition throughout the system. This would have positive effects on both the cost and effectiveness of health care. To avoid undermining the principle of solidarity, there would need to be rules to discourage risk selection, including open enrolment, and measures to discourage self-insurance.

However, there would appear to be formidable political obstacles to structural changes along those lines, and such radical proposals have not yet reached the top of the policy agenda. Meanwhile, the government is continuing with its policy of introducing a succession of more modest reforms discussed earlier, aimed at improving the performance of the health care system.

References

Aiach, P. and Delanoe, J. Y. (1989), "La politique économique du gouvernement socialiste en matière de santé: bilan de cinq années de pouvoir en France, 1981-1986", *Soc. Sci. Med,* Vol. 28, No. 6.

Blendon, R. J., Leitman, R., Morrison, I. and Donelan, K. (1990), "Satisfaction with Health Systems in ten Nations", *Health Affairs,* Summer.

Charlton, J.R.H. and Velez, R. (1986), "Some International Comparisons of Mortality Amenable to Medical Intervention", *British Medical Journal,* Vol. 292, pp. 295-301, 1 February.

CREDES (1989), *L'Évolution des dépenses de santé en France, 1970-1988,* Paris, November.

Commissariat Général du Plan (1989), "Réforme du système de santé: Les projets à l'étude en France", Note for the OECD Working Party on Social Policy, November.

Enthoven, A. (1980), *Health Plan: The Only Practical Solution to the Soaring Cost of Health Care,* Addison-Wesley, Reading, Mass.

Enthoven, A. (1988), *Theory and Practice of Managed Competition in Health Care Finance,* Amsterdam.

Giraud, P. and Launois, R. J. (1985), *Les Réseaux de Soins, Médecine de Demain,* Économica, Paris.

Godt, P. J. (1985), "Doctors and Deficits: Regulating the Medical Profession in France", *Public Administration,* Vol. 63, Summer.

de Kervasdoué, J., Rodwin, V. G. and Stéphan, J. C.(1984), "France: Contemporary Problems and Future Scenarios", in *The End of an Illusion: The Future of Health Policy in Western Industrialised Nations,* de Kervasdoué, J., Kimberly, J. R. and Rodwin, V. G. (eds.), University of California Press.

de Kervasdoué, J. (1988), "L'offre et la demande à l'hôpital", in *Prospective et Santé,* No. 47-48, automne/hiver.

Lacronique, J. F. (1982), "The French Health Care System", in *The Public/Private Mix for Health,* McLachlan, G. and Maynard, A. (eds.), Nuffield Provincial Hospitals Trust, London.

Lacronique, J. F. (1984*a*), "The French Health Services System", in *Reorienting Health Services: Application of a Systems Approach,* Pannenborg, C.O., van der Werff, A., Hirsch, G. B. and Barnard, K. (eds.), NATO conference Series, Plenum Press, New York and London.

Lacronique, J. F. (1984*b*), "Health Services in France", in *Comparative Health Systems,* Raffel, M. W. (ed.), Pennsylvania State University Press.

Lacronique, J. F. (1988), "Technology in France", *International Journal of Technology Assessment in Health Care,* 4, pp. 385-394.

Lanoe, J. L. (1988), *The Financial Constraints of a Health Insurance System*, Working paper for the conference "Medical Consumption and Financial Constraint", Université de l'Europe, London, December.

Launois, R. (1989), "Faut-il avoir peur de Margaret Thatcher?", *Espace Social Européen*, 1 December.

Launois, R., Majnoni d'Intignano, B., Stéphan, J. and Rodwin, V. (1985), "Les réseaux de soins coordonnés (RSC): Propositions pour une réforme profonde du système de santé", *Revue Française des Affaires Sociales*, 39(1), January-March, pp. 37-62.

OECD (1987), *Financing and Delivering Health Care*, Paris.

OECD (forthcoming), *OECD Health Systems: Facts and Trends*, Paris.

de Pouvourville, G. (1986), "Hospital Reforms in France under a Socialist Government", *Milbank Memorial Fund Quarterly*, Vol. 64, No. 3.

Rochaix, L. (1984), "For-Profit Hospitals for Europe: The Case of Britain and France", *Health Policy*, 4, pp. 149-157.

Rodwin, V. G. (1981a), "The Marriage of National Health Insurance and *La médicine libérale:* a costly union", *Milbank Memorial Fund Quarterly*, Vol. 59, No. 1.

Rodwin, V. G. (1981b), "On the Separation of Health Planning and Provider Reimbursement: The United States and France", *Inquiry*, 18, pp. 139-150, Summer.

Rodwin, V. G. (1982), Management without Objectives: The French Health Policy Gamble, in *The Public/Private Mix for Health*, McLachlan, G. and Maynard, A. (eds.), Nuffield Provincial Hospitals Trust, London.

Rodwin, V. G. (1984), "Health Planning under National Health Insurance: France", in *The Health Planning Predicament*, University of California Press, London.

Rozenkier, A. (1990), "The Role of the Social Security System in Providing Social Protection to the Very Old in France", in *The Social Protection of the Frail Elderly*, Studies and Research No. 28, International Social Security Association, Geneva.

Sandier, S. (1989a), "The Payment of Physicians in Selected OECD Countries", OECD, Report for the Working Party on Social Policy, mimeo.

Sandier, S. (1989b), "Quelques aspects du financement des soins médicaux aux États-Unis", *Socio-Économie de la Santé*, CREDES.

Schieber, G. J. and Poullier, J. P. (1989), "International Health Care Expenditure Trends: 1987", *Health Affairs*, Fall, pp. 169-177.

Schieber, G. J., Poullier, J. P. and Greenwald L. M. (1991), "Health Care Systems in Twenty-Four Countries", *Health Affairs*, Fall.

Chapter 5

THE REFORM OF HEALTH CARE IN GERMANY

INTRODUCTION

For 45 years Germany had two health care systems. In the ten *Länder* of the Federal Republic of Germany before unification, the system had experienced no major structural change since its foundations were laid by Bismarck in 1883. However, there was much growth in, and adaptation to, the system during its long history, including some significant reforms in the late 1970s and during the 1980s.

In contrast, following World War II the German Democratic Republic (GDR) before the unification adopted publicly-financed and provided services quite unlike those in the Western *Länder* (Light, 1985). Following the reunification of Germany in October 1990, health service financing and delivery arrangements in the *Länder* of the former GDR are once more being radically reformed to return them to arrangements in force throughout Western *Länder*.

The first part of this chapter describes how health care is financed and provided in the Western *Länder,* and the ways in which the government is involved in regulating and planning services. The second part of the chapter considers the background for recent reforms introduced by the government to the systems in both parts of Germany, with a brief reference to the system in the former German Democratic Republic.

An unusual social experiment – a single country with a single language and a shared history forced to diverge in its political, economic and social institutions for 45 years – provides us with a rare opportunity to compare the performance of health care systems in, respectively, a liberal democracy and a command-and-control state, holding constant the initial conditions and many of the potentially confounding factors (Light, 1985). The growth and performance of both systems are compared, as well as their impact on the health status of the respective populations.

While the most urgent priority which faces policy-makers is the reform of health care in the Eastern *Länder,* there is also a continuing debate about the need for further reforms to the system which has developed in the Western *Länder.* The conclusion considers some outstanding issues and identifies the range of solutions currently being discussed.

HEALTH CARE IN THE WESTERN *LÄNDER*

People in the former Federal Republic of Germany enjoyed access to a generous range and volume of health services, supplied by a mixture of independent and public providers.

Access to services was unhampered by significant direct charges. About 75 % of the population was insured compulsorily, and about 13 % voluntarily with statutory sickness funds. Most of the rest of the population – mainly higher income earners – had private health insurance. In terms of the models described in Chapter 2, the system was dominated by the public contract model, supplemented by the voluntary contract and the voluntary reimbursement models. The bulk of decisions on expenditure were settled between the statutory sickness funds and the providers under arrangements which were both highly decentralised and formalised.

There are about 1 100 autonomous sickness funds. Regional associations of these funds bargain with regional associations of doctors to determine aggregate payments to ambulatory care physicians. In the case of hospitals, representatives of sickness funds negotiate with individual hospitals over rates of payment. These negotiations take place under guidelines for rates of increase of health expenditure set by the Concerted Action Committee (a national body consisting of representatives of interested parties in the health care system which meets twice a year to agree on maximum rates of increases in health expenditure on ambulatory and dental care, pharmaceuticals and other medical supplies). Germany has a federal system of government and the regulation of health services is diffused between the federal, state and local levels.

Chart 5.1 **The system of health care in western Germany: mid-1980s**

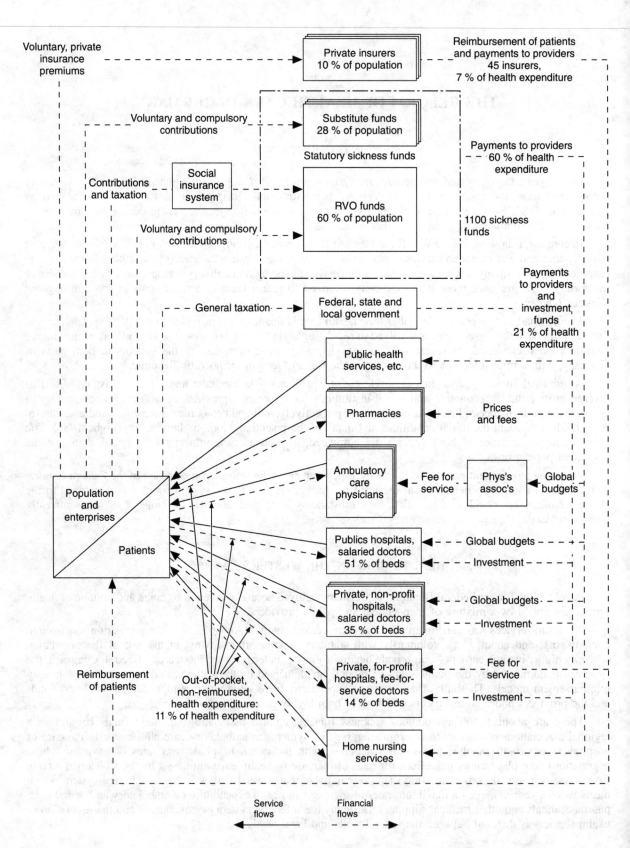

Chart 5.1 summarises some of the main relationships in a simplified form. At the bottom left of the diagram is the population, some of whom become patients during any one year. At the bottom right of the diagram are the providers who supply health services to patients. At the top of the diagram are the third-party payers who collect contributions, premiums or taxes from the population and pay providers or reimburse patients for services delivered. Service flows are shown as solid lines and financial flows are shown as broken lines.

Practically the whole of the population is covered by health insurance. The statutory sickness funds, which cover about 88 % of the population, pay providers directly for the services supplied to their members. The sickness funds can be separated into ''RVO'' (State Insurance Regulation) funds, covering about 60 % of the population, and substitute funds covering about 28 % of the population. The private insurers, which cover about 10 % of the population, provide indemnity payments both in the form of cash reimbursements and in the form of payments to providers. The substitute funds and the private insurers are shown as multiple because there is a certain amount of competition within (and, indeed, between) these segments of the market. The federal, state and local governments are included among the funders because of their role in financing public health services and hospital investment.

In terms of sources of funds, about 60 % of health expenditure is derived from compulsory and voluntary contributions to statutory health insurance, about 21 % is derived from general taxation, about 7 % is derived from private insurance and about 11 % is represented by unreimbursed, out-of-pocket expenditure.

The providers include public health services, pharmacists, physicians in independent practice, public hospitals, private non-profit hospitals, private for-profit hospitals, and home nursing services. The pharmacists, ambulatory care doctors and private for-profit hospitals are shown as multiple as there is usually some competition within these services. Certain other providers such as dentists have been omitted. Sickness funds pay providers by a mixture of global budgets and fee-for-service payments. The bulk of hospital investment in both public and private hospitals is financed by the state governments.

RELATIONSHIP BETWEEN PATIENTS AND PROVIDERS

Most patients can turn to health services knowing that they are amply covered for comprehensive, high-quality care including preventive services, family planning, maternity care, prescription drugs, ambulatory medical care, dental care, transport, hospital in-patient care, home nursing services, rehabilitation services including ''cures'' at spas and income support during sick leave. Public health services and psychiatric services, however, are said to be weak. Nursing homes and homes for the elderly are provided outside the statutory health insurance system by local authorities and voluntary bodies. These are financed mainly by private expenditure, often supported by social assistance.

Patients enjoy free choice of either a general practitioner or a specialist in independent practice. Access to hospital is controlled by ambulatory care doctors and sickness fund patients normally have to go to the nearest hospital with suitable facilities. However, private patients and selected sickness fund patients can be referred outside the area. There is a sharp division between ambulatory care and hospital care. For the most part, hospitals do not offer out-patient care and ambulatory care. Doctors do not generally have access to hospital practice. This system is said to lead to lengthy ''referral chains'', duplication of equipment and repetition of diagnostic tests by different doctors. Ambulatory care practices are well equipped and have ample access to the most advanced diagnostic services. There is a predominance of independent doctors in single practice although partnerships, usually of two doctors in the same speciality, are growing in number.

Patients pay only minor, direct charges for health services under the statutory insurance system. For example, in 1988 prescription charges of DM 2 per person, hospital charges of DM 5 per day were charged for the first 14 days in hospital and charges of DM 5 for non-emergency patient transport. However, these charges were subject to ceilings on total payments and to exemptions, mainly for children and for people with low incomes. Full payments are of course required for over-the-counter medicines and for private medical care, including private rooms in public hospitals. The fees which doctors receive for private patients are higher than those which they receive for sickness fund patients; it is said that there is a corresponding discrimination in the style of service received by the two types of patient (Ade and Henke, 1990). According to OECD figures, the public share of ambulatory care billing was 92 % in 1987 and the public share of in-patient care billing was 98 %.

Four-fifths of the population of the Western *Länder* are covered by the statutory health insurance scheme, of whom two out of five are the dependants of subscribers. About 10 % of the population is fully covered by private insurance – mainly civil servants, the self-employed and high-income earners. Most of the remaining 2 % of the population, including the armed forces, the police and some individuals on social welfare, receive free health services. Less than ¹/₂ % of the population – exclusively well-to-do individuals – has no health insurance.

Membership of sickness funds is split about 85/15 % between compulsory and voluntary members. Membership is compulsory for workers with income below a certain threshold (which was set at DM 54 900 in 1989), for state pensioners, for persons in certain occupations and for certain other persons with modest economic status. Employees with income above the statutory threshold can join the statutory scheme voluntarily as an alternative to private insurance. A majority of those who can insure voluntarily choose a sickness fund in preference to a private insurer because the premiums are usually lower for married couples and families and for older and high-risk workers who have not previously had private insurance. There is consequently selection towards sickness funds.

The statutory scheme is administered by about 1 100 autonomous sickness funds, which are usually controlled by representatives of employers and employees. There are two main types of funds: State Insurance Regulation funds (*RVO-kassen*); and substitute funds (*Ersatzkassen*). The former cater for both blue- and white-collar workers. Some are organised on a local basis, some on an occupational basis and some on an enterprise basis. The latter, which already existed as mutual aid societies when the State scheme was set up, cater mainly for white-collar workers and, because of a certain amount of risk selection, are in a strong position to compete for voluntary members. About half of all members – mainly white-collar workers – can choose their sickness fund. The biggest group of funds are the *RVO-kassen* organised on a local basis (*Ortskrankenkassen*). These funds cater mainly for blue-collar workers and are also obliged to act as a safety net for disadvantaged individuals who do not belong to any group of employees (Eichhorn, 1984).

The sickness funds are required by law to offer a basket of benefits, which has become more generous over time. They are also able to offer additional, optional benefits. The bulk of contributions are made in the form of income-related employers' and employees' contributions (shared 50/50) payable on earnings up to a ceiling. Contributions for state pensioners, the unemployed and the disabled are made from social security funds, but in the case of the pensioners these contributions cover only about half of the cost of benefits. The extra costs are borne by employers and employees and there are cross-subsidies at a federal level between funds to allow for differences in the proportion of retired members. Funds are free to determine their own contribution rates within a guideline (recently 12 %) laid down by law. However, the guideline may be surpassed if a majority of the representatives of the employers and the insured vote for a higher rate. Premiums averaged 12.9 % of gross income in 1988 but, because of different risk structures, ranged widely from 8 to 16 % of income between different funds, with the funds organised on a local basis having the highest average rates. There is considerable competition between the funds for voluntary members. Generally, the funds compete by offering higher optional benefits rather than by lowering premiums.

For the 10 % fully insured privately, this cover is provided by about 45 mainly non-profit insurers. The benefits have to be at least as generous as the minimum basket covered by the statutory scheme. A smaller percentage of Germans take out additional private insurance to supplement the statutory scheme. Deductibles and co-insurance are of increasing importance. The private insurers have agreed collectively to be regulated by a Federal Insurance Office in setting premiums. Premiums on entry depend on: age, sex, risk, numbers of dependants and cost-sharing. They are low for a 20 year old and high for a 50 year old. Subsequently premiums do not vary for age or risk but they can vary for number of dependants and cost-sharing, as well as for rising medical care costs. This system embodies a form of saving and discourages individuals from changing insurer. There is some tax relief on health insurance premiums but this is subject to a ceiling which means, in effect, that marginal additions to premiums are usually financed out of taxed income. Private insurers, unlike sickness funds, provide benefits in the form of reimbursement where physicians' bills are concerned but they usually pay hospital per diem directly to the hospital.

RELATIONSHIP BETWEEN THIRD-PARTY PAYERS AND PROVIDERS

The relationship between the sickness funds and physicians in independent practice is highly formalised. Physicians are, by law, organised into regional and *Länder* associations which assume the duty of making ambulatory medical care available to sickness fund patients and which have considerable powers over individual physicians. The associations are quite separate from doctors' trade unions. All qualified doctors have the right to be admitted to sickness insurance service and, once they are admitted, they must join the physicians' association. The associations bargain with the sickness funds' associations at a sub-*Länder* level over the rate of payment for serving sickness fund patients. They do so in the light of a recommended ceiling on the rate of growth of expenditure on ambulatory physicians' services set by the Concerted Action Committee. The ceiling is set with a view to keeping the contribution rates of insured members constant.

When a local agreement is struck, the sickness funds agree, in effect, to pay a prospective lump sum to the physicians' association. The association itself distributes this sum to individual doctors on the basis of each doctor's workload and according to a fee schedule. The association monitors the quality and volume of services of each physician and, if necessary, applies collective discipline. This system resembles bilateral monopoly at the level of negotiation over the lump sum, although neither the association of sickness funds nor the association of doctors has control over volume.

Volume is decided mainly between patients and individual doctors in a situation where neither has any financial incentive to economise. At the level of the individual doctor, there is competition for volume and income. If one doctor generates, say, 10 % more services, his or her income can rise by a similar amount. However, if all doctors work 10 % harder, fees per item of service must fall by 10 % to keep aggregate expenditure within the agreed total. As a result, each doctor's income will remain unchanged. Similarly, if the number of doctors rises by 10 % and the volume of services per doctor remains unchanged, each doctor's income will fall by 10 % (Brenner, 1989). Recently, the lump sum has been divided into blocks to prevent, say, diagnostic services from taking money from direct patient care (Ade and Henke, 1990).

The fee schedule used by the physicians' association is made up of about 2 500 items of service, a relative points value scale (negotiated nationally and revised infrequently) and a monetary value per point. For example, a telephone conversation with a patient has 80 points, a home visit 360 points and X-rays between 360 and 900 points. The monetary values tend to vary locally and are traditionally higher for the *Ersatzkassen* than for the *RVO-kassen*. They will also move inversely with the number of points billed according to the process previously described. There is a separate, statutory fee schedule for private patients which uses the same relative points value scale. In this case, the fees are about twice the level of those paid by the *RVO-kassen*. Extra billing of private patients (only) is permitted, so long as the relative value scale is used, but this is rare.

Until 1989, there has been relatively little control over expenditure on pharmaceuticals. The wholesale price of drugs has been set unilaterally by the pharmaceutical manufacturers and prescribing has been decided by doctors in the absence of incentives to be economical. There has been only modest cost-sharing by patients. Consequently, there has been only weak price competition. However, there has been a negative list, government-inspired publication of prices for comparable drugs, encouragement of generic prescribing and control of pharmacists' margins.

An interesting variant of these arrangements was the "Bavarian Contract" struck between the sickness funds and the physicians' association in Bavaria in 1979. This allowed for physicians' remuneration in aggregate to rise faster than the negotiated rate provided that savings could be demonstrated in other areas of expenditure under the influence of physicians, such as drug prescribing and hospital referrals (the effects of this contract are discussed later).

There are three main types of hospitals in the Western *Länder* of Germany: public hospitals, which may be owned by federal, *Länder* or local governments accounting for 51 % of beds; private voluntary hospitals, which are often owned by religious organisations, accounting for 35 % of beds; and private, proprietary hospitals, which are often owned by doctors, accounting for 14 % of beds. The first two types of hospital usually have salaried doctors and are paid a per diem rate by the sickness funds which is inclusive of doctors' remuneration. However, the physicians in charge of clinical departments in public hospitals can take private patients. Proprietary hospitals work with doctors who are paid by fee-for-service and they are paid per diem by the sickness funds which are exclusive of doctors' remuneration. Private patients are charged according to the statutory fee schedule for private patients, and usually the doctor must pay some of the fees to the hospital. As has been indicated above, hospital doctors rarely see patients on an out-patient basis and ambulatory care doctors seldom have admitting rights.

Payments to hospitals are made on a dual basis, with operating costs coming mainly from the sickness funds and private insurers and investment expenditure, even in private hospitals, coming mainly from state governments. sickness funds are obliged by law to meet hospitals' historical operating costs but, at the same time, hospitals are obliged to be economical. Since 1986, payments for operating costs have been governed mainly by prospective global budgets negotiated locally by representatives of the sickness funds and individual hospitals. Once again, these negotiations resemble bilateral monopoly. The negotiations are based on a detailed review of operating costs, including physicians' salaries and depreciation, and an expected occupancy rate. They may also be influenced by comparisons with other, efficient hospitals. Negotiations are directed at setting an average daily rate to be used by sickness funds for paying hospitals for each patient day consumed by their members. Charges for private patients are higher, but are based on an average daily rate. Under the global budget, if actual bed days exceed expected bed days during the year, hospitals receive only 25 % of the daily rate for the extra bed days. If actual bed days fall short of expected bed days, the hospital still receives 75 % of the daily rate for the missing bed days. These figures are based on an assumed level for fixed and variable costs during the year. Hospitals can carry over surpluses into subsequent years and must carry losses. If the two parties to the negotiations cannot agree on a prospective budget, the matter is referred to arbitration by a neutral, non-government, price office (Altenstetter, 1987).

There are, however, payments for some high-cost procedures, such as organ transplants, on a cost-per-case basis outside the budget. It is intended to extend these payments to over 100 procedures with a view to: improving the internal transparency of costs; aiding external comparisons: and helping to ensure that payments reflect case mix.

Since 1986, all investments in hospitals accredited under the plans of the *Länder* governments have become the exclusive responsibility of the *Länder*. Private hospitals, including proprietary hospitals, may be included in the plans. Finance is in the form of grants and is written off as soon as the investment is made. In addition, there is still some private investment in proprietary hospitals and this attracts the usual debt charges.

Cost-containment for privately financed health services depends mainly on cost-sharing by the patients, on bonuses for low claims, and by the fact that providers' fees are generally linked to the rates negotiated between the sickness funds and the providers under statutory arrangements. There is little direct negotiation between private insurers and providers and little review of how resources are used.

Quality assurance is becoming a key concern in Germany. A confidential enquiry into perinatal deaths and complications was initiated in Bavaria in 1980, with favourable effects, it has since been extended throughout the Western *Länder*. A similar confidential enquiry into deaths and complications has been established for certain tracer conditions in surgery. Recently, quality assurance was made a statutory requirement for hospitals and the subject of negotiation between sickness funds and the physicians' associations. The law specifies that quality assurance should be done, but not how it should be done. At present, there are no plans to publish information on comparative death and complication rates by hospital. The view seems to be that true comparisons would be technically difficult and that publication would create disincentives for physicians to co-operate in exploring accidents and mistakes.

Public health services are provided mainly by local government. Such services include control of infectious diseases, health education, mother and baby care, and school health services. They are financed by all levels of government and, according to Eichhorn (1984), are seen as something of a poor relation in the health care system.

GOVERNMENT LEGISLATION, REGULATION AND PLANNING

The involvement of government in the Western *Länder* health system has at least three distinct characteristics:
- a strong legal framework set centrally;
- within this, considerable devolution of power and responsibility to sickness funds, physicians' associations and other bodies; and
- diffusion of the remaining government responsibilities between federal, *Länder* and local governments.

Self-government (or *Selbstverwaltung*) is an important principle in the German health care system. The government devolves specified powers and duties to certain regulated but self-governing bodies, including sickness funds and physicians' associations which represent private interest groups, yet have members enrolled on a compulsory basis. These bodies possess considerable autonomy within the framework of regulations set centrally (Stone, 1980).

The principle of devolution of power applies, also, to certain institutions which are designed to regulate, guide and inform the bargaining process arising from countervailing power or bilateral monopoly. The independent arbitration process available to the parties which negotiate hospital budgets falls into this category. So also does the "Concerted Action Committee" set up by the 1977 Cost-Containment Act whose objective is to maintain stability in the rate of health insurance contributions (Henke, 1986). It seems to work mainly through moral persuasion and the incentive the participants have to avoid further cost-containment laws (Schulenburg, 1990*a*). Since 1986, the Concerted Action Committee has been supported by a standing council of expert advisers which has produced a series of influential reports on the shortcomings of the health care system (such as excessive hospital beds) and on suggestions for reforms (such as giving GPs a gatekeeper role in the system and introducing capitation payments for ambulatory care doctors) (Alber, 1989).

Turning to the diffusion of those powers retained by the centre, each level of government has distinct responsibilities.

- The federal government is responsible for: drafting laws; for general policy; and for jurisdiction over the health insurance system.
- The governments of the *Länder* are responsible for approving federal legislation (through their representation in the Upper House); for the local supervision of sickness funds and physicians' associations; for managing *Länder*-owned hospitals, including teaching hospitals; for hospital planning (each *Land* has a plan for controlling capacity in both public and private hospitals); for all investment in hospitals accredited by the *Land* plan; and for regulating standards of medical education and thereby, indirectly, the enrolment of medical students;
- Local governments are responsible for public health services; for managing local hospitals; for investment in local hospitals; and for the management and financing of public nursing homes (which are not covered by the statutory insurance scheme).

These arrangements are not without their tensions. For example, the federal and *Länder* governments may disagree sometimes over general policy. There is often confrontation over hospital expenditure because the federal government tends to identify with the sickness funds, whereas the *Länder* governments have a large stake in the provision of hospital services.

BACKGROUND TO RECENT REFORMS

The Western Länder

The health care system in Germany tends to suffer from a number of problems. One difficulty, which it shares with other systems relying heavily on third-party payment, is a general lack of cost-consciousness. Patients have little financial incentives to limit their demands and providers have few financial incentives to limit the amount of care which they supply. Such competition as does exist tends to be expressed as a struggle to increase volume and quality rather than one to reduce costs. In these circumstances, the mechanism for determining expenditure is transferred to the negotiations between the insurers and the providers. These negotiations tend to take the form of bilateral monopolies.

However, a second difficulty is that, in such markets, the bargaining power of buyers is not always evenly matched with that of sellers. There have been times – such as during the "cost explosion" of the early 1970s – when the providers have had the upper hand. At other times – for example, during the subsequent phase of cost-containment – the balance between the two parties has been more even. Most of the health care reforms which the government introduced from the late 1970s onwards were devoted either to increasing cost-consciousness among consumers and providers, or to strengthening the bargaining power of the sickness funds in their negotiations with providers. In the 1980s the most buoyant programmes in cash terms were pharmaceuticals and hospital expenditure (Schneider, forthcoming).

A further problem concerns the possible inefficient allocation of given resources. Some commentators argue that the combination of a rigid specification by central government of benefits and the incentives contained in the fee schedule combine produce a bias in favour of acute diagnostic and therapeutic procedures and away from personal services, prevention and long-term care. It is also argued that there are excessive number of hospital beds, as well as above average length of stay in hospital.

It was against this background that the federal government began to introduce legislation aimed at containing costs. The 1977 Health Care Containment Act introduced a number of important measures (Stone, 1979) including:

- The principle of income-oriented expenditure policy;
- The Concerted Action conference of interested parties;
- The re-introduction of what amounted to lump-sum prospective budgets for payments by sickness funds to physicians' associations;
- Strengthening of utilisation review of physicians;
- Introduction of, or increases in, cost-sharing for dentures, prescription drugs and patient transport;
- A negative list for drugs; and
- A risk-sharing scheme for pensioners across all sickness funds.

A Supplementary Cost-Containment Act was introduced in 1982 which included, among other measures, further increases in charges for prescription drugs and the publication of the price lists for comparable drugs. A Supplementary Budget Act in 1983 introduced a new charge of DM 5 per day, up to 14 days, for hospital stays a new charge of DM 10 per day for rehabilitation, cures and new prescription charges of DM 2 per drug.

Hospital expenditure had been largely excluded from the 1977 Act. This began to be remedied with the 1982 Hospital Cost-Containment Act (Eichhorn, 1984), the provisions of which included:

– Making hospital daily rates the subject of bargaining between representatives of the sickness funds and the hospitals;
– The involvement of both the associations of sickness funds and the associations of hospitals in the drawing up of State hospital plans.
– Extending the responsibilities of Concerted Action to the hospitals.

Hospital reform was continued with the 1985 Hospital Financing Act and the 1986 Federal Hospital Payment Regulation (Altenstetter, 1987). These provided for:

– Hospital investment to be returned to the *Länder* rather than being shared between the *Länder* and federal governments;
– Prospective global budgets to be introduced for operating costs for each hospital, to be negotiated between representatives of the sickness funds and the hospitals, based on inclusive costs and anticipated occupancy rates;
– Overall, average per diem rates to be set in the light of these costs and comparisons with comparable efficient hospitals;
– Actual payments to be based on 75 % of the agreed daily rate for shortfalls in actual days compared with expected days, and on 25 % of the agreed daily rate for surpluses in actual days compared with expected days;
– Hospitals to be able to carry over surpluses into subsequent years;
– Recourse to neutral arbitration rather than *Länder* government arbitration in the event of disagreement;
– The possibility of special cost-per-case payments for some high-cost procedures;
– Hospitals to begin keeping statistics on the diagnosis, specialty, age and length of stay of their patients with a view to developing cost-per-case pricing at a future date.

The 1986 Need Planning Law enabled physicians' associations and sickness funds to close to newcomers areas with more than a 50 % excess of doctors in certain specialties. In addition, measures were introduced to enable associations and funds to invite doctors to retire early.

Finally, following a jump in average insurance contribution rates from about 11.5 to nearly 13 % in the mid-1980s, which was due both to rising unemployment and to further increases in expenditure, the government introduced a further bulky package of reforms in the 1989 Health Care Reform Act. This is described as the most important statute on the statutory health insurance system since the 1911 Law (Schneider, forthcoming). The Act was aimed both at cost-containment and at financing some selected improvements to benefits. Its contents may be summarised under six headings.

– Requirements for providers to be more economical;
– Revised cost-sharing;
– Changes to benefits;
– Improved regulation of quality, activity, numbers of doctors and conditions of practice;
– Changes to contributions;
– More fundamental reforms to be introduced at a later date.

Requirement for providers to be more economical

The Labour and Social Affairs Ministry introduced fixed payments for drugs with substitutes (no longer on patent) based on the lowest price which would ensure an adequate supply. Fixed reimbursement prices (*Festbestrag*) were to be brought in in stages: first for drugs with the same active ingredient (about a third of the market); then for drugs with therapeutically equivalent ingredients; and, finally for drugs with comparable pharmacological profiles. It was anticipated that, eventually, about 55 % of the market would be directly affected by the new regulations (Jensen, 1990). Once such fixed payments were established for a particular drug, the prescription charge would be abolished. The doctor would remain free to prescribe a product with a price above the fixed payment level but the patient would have to pay the difference. Until the fixed prices were brought in, the prescription charge would be raised from DM 2 to DM 3. These measures were designed to provoke price competition among the pharmaceutical manufacturers. Similar fixed payments based on the lowest viable price for effective products was brought in for other aids and appliances.

- Tighter procedures were introduced for monitoring the prescribing of sickness fund physicians.
- New obligations were introduced for pharmacists to dispense generic equivalents, if prescribed by the doctor.
- Sickness funds were given the freedom to cancel contracts with surplus and uneconomic hospitals.
- Hospitals were obliged to publish price lists and doctors were obliged to consider the cost-effectiveness of their referrals.
- There would be improved co-ordination of in-patient and out-patient care to cut down on unnecessary hospitalisation. This was to be agreed contractually between the sickness funds, hospitals and sickness fund doctors, with recourse to arbitration if necessary.
- Similarly, equipment committees would be set up to reduce duplication of equipment in hospitals and doctors practices.
- New financial incentives would be brought in by *Länder* governments to help cut surplus hospital beds.
- Sickness funds were given the freedom to experiment with innovative ways of providing and paying for services including experimental cost-sharing, no claims bonuses, and new ways of paying providers. The experiments could last up to five years and must be evaluated scientifically.

Revised cost-sharing

- The charge for a hospital day would be increased from DM 5 to DM 10 from 1991.
- Much higher cost-sharing was introduced for patient transport.
- The conditions exempting some patients from charges were revised and new income-related ceilings placed on total charges for any one individual.

Changes to benefits

- Some minor benefits were removed.
- A number of new preventive benefits were introduced – mainly in the form of entitlements to health checks for various age groups.
- Financial support was given to the carers of the long-term sick. The sickness funds would pay for: up to four weeks' holiday for family carers beginning from 1989; and a long-term care allowance of either DM 400 per month for the family carer or DM 750 per month for professional nursing services, designed to purchase up to 25 hours of care, from 1991.

Improved regulation

- Quality assurance programmes were to be introduced for both ambulatory care and hospital doctors following negotiations between sickness fund and the physicians' associations. The method of quality assurance was to be left to the interested parties but it was envisaged, for example, that utilisation review involving random samples of 2 % of ambulatory care doctors each quarter would be instituted.
- The medical examiner service would be transformed into an independent medical advisory service for the sickness funds.
- The *Länder* governments were urged to act further to reduce, by indirect means, the intake to medical schools.
- There would be tightening of the conditions for doctors to be admitted to practice with the sickness funds.

Changes to contributions

- An income limit was introduced for compulsory health contributions by blue-collar workers, giving them the same conditions as salaried workers.
- Pensioners' contributions were to be raised to the same average level as workers' contributions (6.4 %) beginning in 1989.
- Contributions for children insured in the public system by privately insured parents would be doubled.

More fundamental reforms

It was envisaged that more fundamental reforms, involving a modernisation of the organisational structures of the sickness funds, would be introduced at a later date. The aim would be to reduce differentials in contribution rates, to remove distortions to competition and to abolish inequalities in the treatment of manual workers and salaried employees. In May 1992, the Health Ministry decided to introduce a new set of reforms (Schneider, forthcoming).

The Eastern Länder

Prior to reunification, the German Democratic Republic had centralised, integrated, publicly financed and provided health services. The great bulk of pharmaceutical, ambulatory medical care and hospital services were organised under the State and were provided free of charge to patients. There was emphasis on ambulatory health centres (or polyclinics) and on occupational health services. Services were funded by a mixture of payroll taxes and general taxes. Although patients could choose their doctor, the doctors themselves were salaried and were very much under the control of the State. There was only a very small private sector (see Chart 5.2 which sets out the key features of the health care system of the former German Democratic Republic in 1989).

In the negotiations which led to the reunification, it was decided to put the health system on the same financial and organisational basis as that of Western *Länder* as quickly as possible. The main changes proposed are as follows:

– On January 1, 1991 a complete network of *Ortskrankenkassen* (local sickness funds) came into operation in the Eastern *Länder*. Other sickness funds will be free to set up if they wish.

Chart 5.2 **Key relationships in the health care system of the former German Democratic Republic**

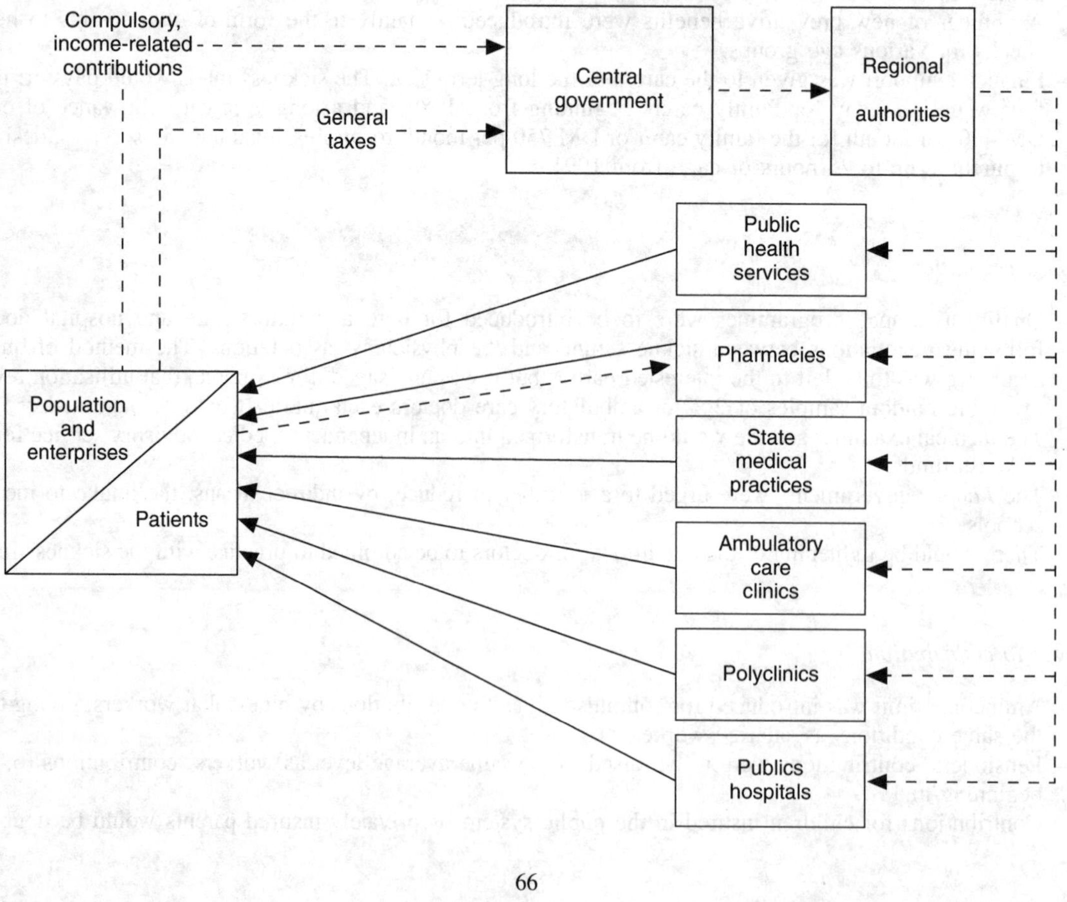

- The great majority of the population was insured compulsorily because of their income levels.
- The contribution rate to all sickness funds was set at 12.8 % (the average rate in the Western *Länder*), for at least a year.
- The aim is for expenditure to balance income. This will be facilitated by setting average fees and charges in the Eastern *Länder* at 45 % of the level prevailing in the Western *Länder* (reflecting the estimated difference in the current standards of living in the two parts of Germany).
- In the case of pharmaceuticals, although prices will be homogeneous in the entire country, in the Eastern *Länder* there will be a larger discount for the mandatory sickness funds than in the Western *Länder*. In fact, the pharmaceutical industry has undertaken to share with the public sector, to a limited extent, any deficits incurred by the funds because of high prices and or increases in consumption of pharmaceuticals.
- On the delivery side, polyclinics and group practices remain popular with many doctors in the Eastern *Länder,* especially older doctors and women who wish to continue working part-time. They also remain popular with a majority of patients. Consequently, polyclinics remain in operation, but will be reviewed after five years.
- The doctors will be able to chose between continuing salaried service, and fee-for-service payment as in the Western *Länder*. This is presenting difficulties because fees in the the Western *Länder* are inclusive of practice expenses whereas salaries in the Eastern *Länder* exclude the overheads of polyclinics.
- A need has been identified for up to DM 20bn of investment in buildings and equipment to bring standards up to those in the Western *Länder*.

PERFORMANCE OF THE TWO SYSTEMS COMPARED

The Western Länder

To summarise: most Germans living in the Western *Länder* are covered either by statutory or private health insurance which offers access to a high level of health care and ensures that, for the most part, they have little incentive to economise. Consumers have free choice among ambulatory care physicians but most do not have free choice of insurer. Providers have considerable autonomy and financial incentives to expand care but when it comes to payment they face the associations of autonomous sickness funds, which are charged with stabilizing the contribution rates of their members. The formalised and regulated bargaining which ensues resembles bilateral monopoly, although the sickness funds cannot control volume. On many occasions in the past, the bargaining has favoured the providers. However, for over a decade the federal government has sought to tip the balance towards the sickness funds by legislating for the promulgation of agreed national guidelines on rates of growth of expenditure, for fixed prospective budgets for physicians' associations and hospitals, and for independent arbitration on hospital rates. On the whole, there has been little price competition, as opposed to quality competition, but steps have been taken recently towards encouraging price competition in the supply of pharmaceuticals and hospital services.

The federal government was successful in stabilizing the share of health expenditure in GDP following the cost explosion of the early 1970s. The share had leaped from 5.5 % of GDP in 1970 to 7.8 % of GDP in 1975. According to OECD figures, in 1980 health's share was 8.5 %, in 1988 8.9 % and in 1990 8.1 %. Measured in dollars, converted at purchasing power parity exchange rates, health expenditure per capita was $1 093 in 1987, close to that for France and the Netherlands but almost 50 % more than that in the United Kingdom. Health expenditure per capita was almost exactly at the level which would be predicted by a regression line associating per capita health expenditure with per capita GDP for all OECD countries (Schieber and Poullier, 1989).

There are suggestions, however, that per capita health expenditure may lie above the regression line suggested by the OECD figures. Some commentators report that health expenditure, excluding transfer payments, represented between 9 and 10 % of GDP (or GNP) between 1975 and 1984 (see Reinhardt, 1981; Altenstetter, 1986; Henke, 1988 and 1990). Also, it seems that Germany is one of the OECD countries whose health system accounts comprise little expenditure on nursing homes.

As might be expected, expenditure on privately insured services has risen more rapidly than expenditure on publicly insured services during the era of cost-containment. The private share of expenditure went up from 18 % in 1977 to 22 % in 1989 (Schneider, forthcoming).

In the past couple of years, the federal government has been successful in meeting the financial objectives which it set in the 1989 Health Care Reform Act. The rate of growth of expenditure by the sickness funds fell from 5.8 % per annum in 1988 to 3 % per annum in 1989. About 300 sickness funds have been able to lower their contribution rates and, at the time of writing it was hoped that average contribution rates would fall to 12.6 % in 1992 (from about 12.9 % in 1988) instead of rising to 13.5 % in the absence of the reforms. The reported share of GDP devoted to health expenditure fell from 8.9 in 1988 to 8.1 % in 1990. Among other measures, four uneconomic hospitals were closed and 20 more closures have been planned. The introduction of fixed payments for drugs has been particularly successful. In the first year, prices of drugs included in the scheme fell by 21 %, whereas the prices of drugs outside the scheme rose by 2 %, most producers of the therapeutic classes covered by the scheme lowered their prices to the reimbursement ceiling (Schneider, forthcoming). There was relatively little sign of consumers being willing to pay for branded products.

Turning to volume and price, the Western *Länder* have more acute beds per thousand (7.6), more consultations with GPs per capita (10.8) and more medicines prescribed outside hospitals per capita (11.2) than the other six countries in this study (see table 10.2 in Chapter 10). Moreover, although average hospital length of stay has been falling, it is the longest average in acute hospital (13.5 days in 1986). There are no reports of hospital waiting lists. The ratio of physicians per thousand population (at 2.8) is above the average of the seven countries. Projections suggest that physician numbers will rise by a further 50 % by 2000 (Brenner, 1989). The ratio of physicians' income to average wages is unusually high but has been falling with increasing numbers of physicians (Sandier, 1989). Average drug prices have been estimated to be the highest in the European Community (SNIP, 1988).

There were disappointing results from the 1979 Bavarian Contract which was aimed at rewarding ambulatory care physicians for cutting expenditure on prescribing and hospital referrals. Overall, it seems that there was relatively little substitution of physician services for prescribing and hospital referrals and no savings in costs. One explanation is that the financial incentives in the scheme were designed to work only at an aggregate level, giving individual physicians little motive to make economies. Also, in the case of hospital expenditure, the existence of retrospective, per diem, cost reimbursement at the time the Contract was signed, meant that any reduction in admissions could be countered by hospitals through rising length of stay or the concentration of fixed costs (Jurgen and Potthoff, 1987).

What has been the impact of a high and growing level of health expenditure on the health status of the population? This is difficult to assess because many other factors, not least a high and growing standard of living generally, influenced health. However, it is worth reporting that in 1987 the Western *Länder* were a middle-ranking OECD country in terms of male and female life expectancy at birth. It was a better than middling country in terms of perinatal mortality in 1989, having moved sharply up the international league table from a below middle-ranking position in the 1960s. There was a marked improvement in perinatal mortality in the 1970s from 2.6 % of births in 1970 to 1.2 % of births in 1980. This was followed by a further sharp improvement to 0.7 by 1988, which exceeded that for the other six countries in this study for which we have data. Germany now has one of the lowest perinatal mortality rates in the OECD. Some epidemiologists in Germany believe that the improvements in the 1980s were due, at least in part, to the introduction of quality assurance programme in hospital obstetrics departments.

Finally, a recent survey which looked at consumer satisfaction with health systems in ten countries (Blendon *et al.,* 1990) suggested that the population of the Western *Länder* were relatively satisfied. Germany ranked third equal (with France) in the percentage of respondents who thought that only "minor changes" were needed in their health care systems.

The Eastern Länder

While the full history of the social "experiment" in the German Democratic Republic has yet to be written, the overwhelming verdict among the people of both sides of the former dividing line is that "socialism did not work". Not only was there more personal freedom for most of the people for most of the time in the Western *Länder* than in the Eastern *Länder,* standards of living also rose much more quickly in the Federal Republic. Looking in particular at health care in the former Democratic Republic, however, what evidence is there that the system did not work?

Statistics on health expenditure in the former Democratic Republic are not easy to come by and raise more problems of reliability and comparability. Expenditure on medical care was reported at 5.5 % of national income in 1980 compared with a figure of 8.5 % for the Western *Länder* in the same year (Ministry of Health, GDR, 1981). The ratio of GNP per capita in the Eastern *Länder* compared to this of the Western *Länder* has been variously estimated at figures ranging from 0.56 to 0.81 (Lohmann, 1986). Clearly, the German Democratic Republic had a standard of living well below that of the Federal Republic of Germany before reunification and spent less, as a proportion, on health services. It must, therefore, have had much lower health expenditure per capita.

However, in terms both of the real resources devoted to health and health service activities, the two countries seem to have been fairly similar. According to the World Health Organisation (1988) the Democratic Republic had 2.3 physicians per thousand in 1985 compared with 2.6 in the Federal Republic. In 1977, the Democratic Republic was reported as having 10.6 hospital beds per thousand compared with 11.8 in the Federal Republic and both regions had similar levels of dentists and pharmacists per thousand (Lohmann, 1986). Hospital length of stay was reported as similar in the two countries (Rosenberg and Ruban, 1986). Given that hospital beds per thousand were similar, this suggests that admission rates were not very different. Finally, consultation rates with doctors seem to have been similar, at 9 per person in the Democratic Republic in 1976 (Rosenberg and Ruban, 1986) and 10.9 per person in the Federal Republic in 1975. If the Eastern *Länder* enjoyed a similar volume of health services to those of the Western *Länder,* with much lower health expenditure per capita, then the prices of health services must have been much lower in the German Democratic Republic.

Turning to health status, the reported life expectancy at birth in the Eastern *Länder,* 69.9 for men and 76.0 for women in 1987, was not far behind that of the Western *Länder* at 72.2 for men and 78.9 for women in 1987. The infant mortality rate, 7.2 % in 1950, had fallen to 0.92 % by 1986. Although that rate was still above that of the Western *Länder* in 1986 (0.85) the fall since 1950 (when it was 5.6 in the Western *Länder*) is larger.

On the basis of its official figures, the former Democratic Republic exhibited a respectable health record for a country with its standard of living. Improvements to health status seem to have kept up, more or less, with those in the Western *Länder* despite the fact that the standard of living grew much more slowly in the East. Given that the crude volume of some of the major health services was similar in the two countries, it could be argued that the system was at least as effective as that in the Western *Länder.* It is clear that the Eastern *Länder* lacked much of the equipment and many of the drugs available in the Western *Länder.* However, it seems that doctors in the Eastern *Länder* received training at least as long as that in the Western *Länder.* Moreover, Light (1985) has argued that whereas the Eastern *Länder* system suppressed some aspects of physicians' autonomy and relied on centralised management, it also: introduced integration of hospital and ambulatory care; linked health with housing, workplace and schools; and placed emphasis on prevention (starting with compulsory comprehensive vaccination of children). By contrast, whereas the Western *Länder* health care system emphasized the autonomy of physicians, sickness funds and patients, and introduced a wealth of curative, high-technology medicine, it preserved doctor-induced demarcation between hospitals and ambulatory care and neglected some preventive medicine. Although there are too many factors at work here to be sure of causation, it is not obvious that the strengths lay exclusively in the Western *Länder.*

CONCLUSION: A CONTINUING DEBATE

The Western Länder

The durability of the system of health care in the Western *Länder* is a testament to its many strengths. The system has achieved high and equitable standards of health care, while preserving patient choice and provider autonomy. There has been striking success in reducing perinatal mortality in recent years. The reforms aimed at containing costs have stabilized health expenditure's share of GDP. The system has also performed well in an international survey which measured satisfaction levels with health care systems.

These objectives have been achieved in a predominantly publicly financed system without significant cost-sharing or central intervention of the command and control type. It is true that there has been a strong and effective central government policy on the rate of growth of health expenditure and planning of hospital facilities by the *Länder* governments. However, apart from this, the system relies mainly on self-regulation by establishing a balance of negotiating power between autonomous sickness funds and providers, and by allowing consumer choice to determine much of the flow of funds in ambulatory care. More recently, there have been some careful moves in the direction of increasing competition among hospitals. Generally, mixed systems of reimbursement prevail which provide both baseline expenditure and rewards for productivity, within global budgets.

However, although the government has had much success in containing costs over the past decade and a half, there are still some adverse pressures. To some extent, these are a result of factors outside the control of government, such as the ageing of the population. Germany is facing a marked deterioration in the dependency ratio over the next four decades which will present financial problems for the pay-as-you-go social security and the health care system (Schulenburg, 1990*b*). To some extent, the pressures which the system faces are attributable to factors which might be amenable to further reform. These include apparent overcapacity in hospital, continuing provider incentives to escalate the volume and quality of care and a low level of competition among insurers and some providers.

There also appears to be some concern in the German literature about efficiency and cost-effectiveness in the health care system. Some commentators argue that there is a relative over-production of high-technology, curative, somatic medical care and a relative underproduction of preventive, psychiatric care and long-term care. This seems to be the result of a combination of rigidly specified benefits under the public scheme and the nature and structure of the fee-for-service incentives for doctors and other providers. Hospital efficiency has come under particular scrutiny (Ballay, 1990). The average length of stay is regarded as excessive, and is likely to stem from: overcapacity in beds, the past and continuing role accorded to per diem payments; the sharp separation between ambulatory and hospital care; the lack of care facilities for sick and elderly people in the community and the dual hospital financing system which means that the *Länder* governments, responsible for planning and investment in capacity, are not responsible for running costs.

Furthermore, there are mixed feelings about the rate of growth in the number of doctors. Projections suggest that the numbers will rise by 50 % by 2000. Whereas a further increase is likely to help any competitive strategy and further reduce the relative income of physicians, it is also likely to generate induced demand for services under fee-for-service remuneration (Schulenburg, 1990*b*).

Equity still remains a problem in that there is not always equal treatment for equal need. Generally, white-collar workers have more choice in health care than blue-collar workers, especially if they are above the income ceiling for compulsory insurance. Meanwhile, compulsorily insured individuals, with the same risk characteristics and income, may find themselves paying different contributions simply because they are obliged to belong to sickness funds whose memberships have different risk profiles.

Finally, some critics argue that sickness funds are overregulated and have inadequate incentives to act as efficient buyers on behalf of their members. There is little, if any, competitive pressure on the funds, and there is some disillusionment with the quality of control exerted by the boards which represent employers and employees.

The Eastern Länder

The system of health care in the Eastern *Länder,* now being partly dismantled, could also lay some claims to past successes. Despite relatively low expenditure and poor facilities, the system helped to bring about improvement to health indicators such as infant mortality. Well-trained and adequately salaried doctors were apparently capable of delivering a high proportion of the available range of effective medical care with relatively few drugs and vaccines and with relatively simple facilities and equipment. The system probably benefited from multi-specialty group practice and good integration between ambulatory and hospital care. However, physical standards were low, there was a lack of high technology, doctors had little autonomy and such patient choice as existed was not translated into financial incentives for providers. The whole system is discredited by its association with the former Democratic Republic. There has been a conclusive decision by the German governement to abandon this experiment with an autocratic, integrated health care model in favour of the liberal, contract model devised by Bismarck.

POTENTIAL SOLUTIONS

The most urgent priority following reunification is the reform of health care in the Eastern *Länder* to bring it into line with that in the Western *Länder*. The government decided to reintroduce sickness funds in the Eastern *Länder,* to set contribution levels at the same average level as in Western *Länder* and to begin with fees and prices at about half the level of those in the Western *Länder*. The ultimate fate of polyclinics and salaried medical practice in the Eastern *Länder* is not yet clear. A more pluralistic system of health care than that which prevailed in the Western *Länder* may eventually emerge from the reunification of the two parts of the country.

Meanwhile, the debate continues about the need for further reforms to the system. Under discussion are new arrangements for financing long-term care involving either; the introduction of a mandatory, funded scheme for private insurance offering a cash benefit which would pay for nursing home care or domiciliary care; or the introduction of a new, long-term care benefit covering similar services in kind to be administered (separately) by the sickness funds with compulsory contributions on a pay-as-you-go basis. Reorganisation of the sickness funds is also on the policy agenda, with a view to reducing differentials in contribution rates, removing distortions to competition and abolishing inequities in the treatment between manual workers and salaried employees. There are signs that these objectives will be achieved from the outset in this Eastern *Länder*. Proposals for introducing a gatekeeper role for GPs and capitation payments in place of fee-for-service payments for ambulatory care doctors have been put forward by the group of experts which advises the Concerted Action Committee.

70

Finally, some independent experts have floated ideas about more radical structural reforms, involving fully competitive insurance and provider markets (Gitter *et al.,* 1989; Jacobs, 1989). The systems being proposed are aimed at combining the "solidarity" principle for health insurance with a competitive market both for insurance and for health care itself. They bear some resemblance to the Dekker proposals in the Netherlands (see Chapter 7) and to the ideas put forward for managed competition in France (see Chapter 4, Launois *et al.,* 1985). However, these proposals have not yet been spelled out as clearly as those in the Netherlands and, as in France, there is no sign at present that they will be taken up by the government.

References

Ade, C. and Henke, K. D. (1990), "Medical Manpower Policies in the Federal Republic of Germany", University of Hannover, typescript, November.

Alber, J. (1989), "Structural Reforms in the West German Health Care System", paper prepared for a Conference on Structural Reforms of National Health Care Systems, University of Maastricht, December 8-9.

Alber, J. (1990), "Characteristics of the West German Health Care System in Comparative Perspective", in E. Kolinsky (Ed.), *The Federal Republic – Forty Years on,* Berg, Oxford, New York.

Altenstetter, C. (1986), "Reimbursement Policy of Hospitals in the Federal Republic of Germany", *International Journal of Health Planning and Management"*, Vol. 1, pp. 189-211.

Altenstetter, C. (1987), "An End to a Consensus on Health Care in the Federal Republic of Germany?", *Journal of Health Politics, Policy and Law,* Vol. 12, No. 3, Fall.

Ballay, U. (1990), "Waste for Profit", *The Health Services Journal,* January 25.

Beske, F. (1982), "Expenditures and Attempts of Cost-Containment in the Statutory Health Insurance System of the Federal Republic of Germany", in *The Public/Private Mix for Health,* eds. McLachlan, G. and Maynard, A. The Nuffield Provincial Hospitals Trust.

Beske, F. (1988), "Federal Republic of Germany", in *The International Handbook of Health-Care Systems,* ed. Saltman, R.B., Greenwood Press.

Blendon, R.J., Leitman, R., Morrison, I. and Donelan, K. (1990), "Satisfaction with Health Systems in Ten Nations", *Health Affairs,* Summer.

Brenner, G. (1989), "Cost-Controlling Measures in Out-Patient Medical Care in the Federal Republic of Germany", paper presented to the First European Conference on Health Economics, Barcelona, September.

Breyer, F. (1989), "Distributional Effects of Coinsurance Options in Social Health Insurance Systems", paper presented to the First European Conference on Health Economics, Barcelona, September.

Eichhorn, S. (1984), "Health Services in the Federal Republic of Germany", in *Comparative Health Systems,* Ed. Raffel, M. W., Pennsylvania State University.

Enthoven, A. C. (1988), *Theory and Practice of Managed Competition in Health Care Finance,* Amsterdam.

Glaser, W. A. (1983), "Lessons from Germany: Some Reflections Occasioned by Schulenburg's Report", *Journal of Health Politics, Policy and Law,* Vol. 8, No. 2, Summer.

Glaser, W. A. (1987), *Paying the Hospital,* Jossey-Bass Inc., San Francisco.

Gitter, W., Hauser, H., Henke, K. D., Knappe, E., Manner, L., Neubauer, G., Oberender, P. and Sieben, G. (1989), *Structural Reform of the Statutory Health Insurance System,* Scientific Study Group "Health Insurance", Universität Bayreuth, June.

Godt, P. J. (1987), "Confrontation, Consent, and Corporatism: State Strategies and the Medical Profession in France, Great Britain, and West Germany", *Journal of Health Politics, Policy and Law,* Vol. 12, No. 3, Fall.

Goebel, W. (1989), "Reform of Health Services in the Federal Republic of Germany", *International Social Security Review,* 4/89.

Henke, K. D. (1986), "A 'Concerted' Approach to Health Care Financing in the Federal Republic of Germany", *Health Policy,* Vol. 6, pp. 341-351.

Henke, K. D. (1988), *The Health Care System of the Federal Republic of Germany,* Discussion Paper No. 119, Universität Hannover, April.

Henke, K. D. (1990), Comments on a Report by Jönsson, B., in *Health Care Systems in Transition,* OCDE, Paris.

Henke, K. D. (1990), "The Federal Republic of Germany", in *Advances in Health Economics and Health Services Research,* Supplement 1: *Comparative Health Systems,* JAI Press Inc.

Jacobs, K. (1989), ''Elements of Competition in the Statutory Health Insurance the Case of the Federal Republic of Germany'', paper presented to the First European Conference on Health Economics, Barcelona, September.

Jensen, A. (1990), *Price Ceilings for Pharmaceuticals – Recent Experiences with a New Instrument in Health Politics,* Bundesverband der Betriebskrankenkassen, Germany.

Jurgen, J. and Potthoff, P. (1987), ''Cost-Containment in a Statutory Health Insurance Scheme by Substitution of Outpatient for Inpatient Care? The Case of the Bavarian Contract'', *Health Policy,* Vol. 8, pp. 153-169.

Klinkmuller, E. (1986), ''The Medical-Industrial Complex'', in *Political Values and Health Care: the German Experience,* eds. Light, D.W. and Scholar, A., The MIT Press.

Launois, R., Majnoni d'Intignano, B., Stéphan, J. et Rodwin V. (1985), ''Les réseaux de soins coordonnés (RSC): proposition pour une réforme profonde du système de santé'', *Revue Française des Affaires Sociales,* 39(1), January-March, pp. 37-62.

Leidl, R. (1983), ''The Hospital Financing System of the Federal Republic of Germany'', *Effective Health Care,* Vol. 1, No. 3.

Light, D.W. (1985), ''Values and Structure in the German Health Care Systems'', *Milbank Memorial Fund Quarterly/Health and Society,* Vol. 63, No. 4.

Lohmann, U. (1986), ''Sociological Portrait of the Two Germanies'', in *Political Values and Health Care: the German Experience,* Ed. Light, D. W. and Schuller, A., The MIT Press.

Ministry of Health (GDR), 1981, *Health Care in the German Democratic Republic,* Berlin, May.

Neubauer, G. and Unterhuber, H. (1985), ''Failures of the Hospital Financing System of the Federal Republic of Germany and Reform Proposals'', *Effective Health Care,* Vol. 2, No. 4.

Neuhaus, R. and Schrader, W. F. (1985), ''Planning and Management of Public Health in the Federal Republic of Germany'', *Health Policy,* Vol. 5, pp. 99-109.

OECD (1987), *Financing and Delivering Health Care,* Paris.

OECD (forthcoming), *OECD Health Systems: Facts and Trends,* Paris.

Reinhardt, U. E. (1981), ''Health Insurance and Health Policy in the Federal Republic of Germany'', *Health Care Financing Review,* Vol. 3, No. 2, December.

Rosenberg, P. and Ruban, M. E. (1986), ''Social Security and Health Care Systems'', in *Political Values and Health Care; the German Experience,* Ed. Light, D. W. and Schuller, A., The MIT Press.

Sahmer, S. (1989), ''Public and Private Health Insurance'', paper presented to the Conference on Health Care in Europe after 1992, Rotterdam, October.

Sandier, S. (1990), ''Health Services Utilization and Physician Income Trends'', in *Health Care Systems in Transition,* OCDE, Paris.

Schieber, G. J. and Poullier, J.-P. (1989), ''International Health Care Expenditure Trends'', *Health Affairs,* Fall.

Schicke, R. K. (1988), ''Trends in the Diffusion of Selected Medical Technology in the Federal Republic of Germany'', *International Journal of Technology Assessment in Health Care,* Vol. 4, pp. 395-405.

Schneider, M. (forthcoming), ''Evaluation of Cost-Containment Acts in the Federal Republic of Germany'', in OECD, *Health: Quality and choice.*

Schulenburg, J.-M.G. (1983), ''Report from Germany: Current Conditions and Controversies in the Health Care System'', *Journal of Health Politics, Policy and Law,* Vol. 8, No. 2, Summer.

Schulenburg, J.-M.G. (1990*a*), ''Health Care in the '90s: a Report from Germany'', typescript, University of Hannover.

Schulenburg, J.-M.G. (1990*b*), ''The German Health Care System from an Economic Perspective'', typescript, University of Hannover, July.

Schulz, R. and Harrison, S. (1986), ''Physician Autonomy in the Federal Republic of Germany, Great Britain and the United States'', *International Journal of Health Planning and Management,* Vol. 2.

SNIP, Syndicat national des industries pharmaceutiques (1988), *Les prix des spécialités pharmaceutiques remboursables dans la Communauté européenne,* Paris.

Stone, D. A. (1979), ''Health Care Cost-Containment in West Germany'', *Journal of Health Politics, Policy and Law,* Vol. 4, No. 2, Summer.

Stone, D. A. (1980), ''National Health Care in the Federal Republic of Germany'', *The Limits of Professional Power,* University of Chicago Press.

WHO (World Health Organisation) (1988), *World Health Statistics Annual,* Genève.

Zweifel, P. (1987), ''Bonus Systems in Health Insurance: a Microeconomic Analysis'', *Health Policy,* Vol. 7, pp. 273-288.

Chapter 6

THE REFORM OF THE HEALTH SYSTEM IN IRELAND

INTRODUCTION

The Irish health care system contains a unique combination of public and private institutions. This chapter describes the way health care is financed and delivered in Ireland and the reforms to the system in the 1980s. It goes on to discuss the recent growth and performance of the system and some of its strengths and weaknesses.

Although voluntary insurance plays an important role, the main source of finance is general taxation and, as a consequence, the government has considerable discretion over the rate of growth of expenditure. Following rapid growth in health expenditure during the 1970s and a deterioration in the Irish economy, the government decided to make sharp cuts in real health expenditure in the 1980s. This led to mounting public concern and controversy. In response to this, the government appointed a Commission on Health Funding in June 1987 which reported in September 1989 with a number of proposals for major reforms, put into effect in 1991. The chapter concludes by describing and assessing the recommendations of this Commission.

HEALTH CARE SYSTEM DESCRIBED

So far as financing of health care is concerned, the Irish system is an example of the social assistance model. That is to say, the poorest one-third of the population (category I) has been given full eligibility for free health services funded out of general taxation. Until 1989, half of the population with middle incomes has been given more limited eligibility for free services, and the richest 15 % has been given still more limited eligibility. Within the public system, general practitioner services are supplied under the contract model, and hospital services are supplied under the integrated model. Because of limited eligibility, private expenditure plays an important role in the system. Private health insurance is available on a voluntary basis, and has been taken up by about 30 % of the population. It is available, however, only from a single, public insurer, the Voluntary Health Insurance Board. On the delivery side, there is a mix of public and private provision with independent general practitioners and a mix of public, voluntary and private hospitals.

The main features of the system can be depicted diagramatically (see Chart 6.1). At the bottom left of the diagram is the population, most of whom become patients in any one year. At the bottom right of the diagram are the providers who supply health services to patients. At the top of the diagram are the third-party payers. Service flows are shown as solid lines and financial flows as broken lines.

The providers have been separated into: public health services, pharmacists (retail chemists), general practitioners, voluntary general hospitals (some of whose beds are private), public general hospitals (some of whose beds are private), public special hospitals (for geriatric, mentally handicapped and psychiatric patients), community health services (including home nursing, dental, aural and ophthalmic services), and private general and psychiatric hospitals. There are considerable flows of direct payments from patients to providers.

The third-party payers have been separated into the Department of Health and the Voluntary Health Insurance Board. Also shown are the health boards (of which there are eight) which fund and manage public services locally, and the General Medical Services (Payments) Board which funds general practitioners and pharmacists, for Category I patients, on behalf of the health boards. Most of the services which are funded publicly are funded through the health boards, with the exception of the voluntary hospitals which are funded directly by the Department of Health.

The financial flows usually involve separate, recurrent expenditure and capital grants, with the exception of those to independent practitioners, such as the pharmacists and GPs, which involve fees and payments which cover annuitised reimbursement for capital. Until recently, the Voluntary Health Insurance Board reimbursed its members for medical care bills on a charge basis for services covered under its policies. However, the Board is

Chart 6.1 **The system of health care in Ireland**

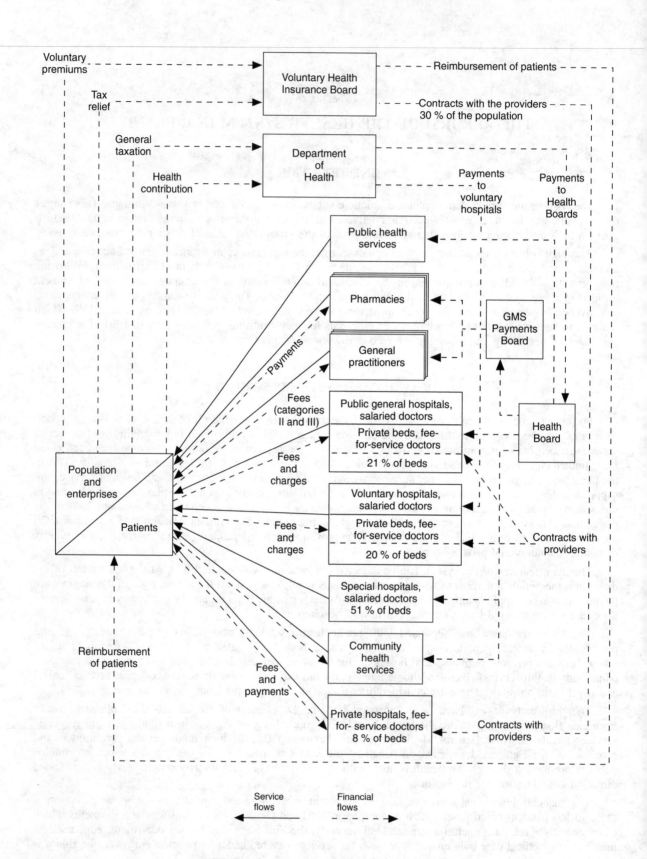

now capping payments and paying most providers directly, with the result that some patients are themselves having to cover the extra billing.

RELATIONSHIP BETWEEN PATIENTS AND PROVIDERS

Everybody enjoys eligibility for a full range of modern health services, but the terms on which access to some of these services takes place varies according to eligibility and insurance coverage. The main distinction is between public and private patients. For example, about 40 % of consultations with GPs and 25 to 30 % of in-patient episodes in general hospitals are private (that is to say, fee-paying). The public share of ambulatory care billing is one of the lowest in the OECD (Poullier, 1990, Table 19). Clearly, access to private care depends on either ability to pay or insurance cover, which tends to be taken out mainly by middle and higher income groups.

All patients can choose their GP, but whereas private patients may switch doctors at will, public patients must register with a GP who participates in the public scheme and must apply to the Health Board for a change of doctor. GPs act as gatekeepers and they usually work on their own rather than in group practices. Tussing (1985) has estimated that 72 % of hospital expenditure and 98 % of the cost of prescription medicines is instigated directly or indirectly by GPs. He also observed that GPs in Ireland have much higher hospital referral rates than their counterparts in England. This may be because their practices are often single-handed. So far as expenditure is concerned, hospitals dominate and more than 60 % of doctors work in hospitals, either as consultants or as junior doctors. If the GP issues a pharmaceutical prescription, the patient usually takes it to a retail chemist for the drug to be dispensed, but in rural areas doctors are allowed to do their own dispensing. Private patients usually pay for prescriptions out of their own pockets (for the exceptions, see below) but Category I patients are entitled to free drugs. GPs' fees for private patients are set by the market, although there is no overt competition over price. Pharmaceutical prices are controlled, even for private patients.

Eligibility and insurance cover determine the terms on which access to health care takes place. Until recently, there were three categories of eligibility:

Category I: Adult persons and their dependants who are judged to be unable to arrange GP services for themselves and their dependants without undue hardship. In practice, they represent about 37 % of the population. They are eligible for the full range of publicly financed health services free of charge and they are given medical cards as evidence of this. The issue of a medical card depends mainly on a means test but chronic illness may also be taken into account.

Category II: All remaining adult persons and their dependants with income below a certain threshold (£16 000 in the 1988-1989 tax year). They represent about 48 % of the population. They are eligible for all publicly financed health services except free GP services and free prescribed medicines below a certain threshold level of expenditure each month, or in the case of certain chronic illnesses. In addition, they must pay £10 for the first hospital out-patient visit for any condition and £10 per day for the first ten days of public in-patient care in any one year.

Category III: Adult persons and their dependants with income above the threshold of £16 000, mentioned above. They represented in 1988 about 15 % of the population. In addition to the exclusions mentioned for Category II, they were not eligible for free hospital consultants' services or for free maternity and infant welfare services in the community. In addition, like Category II patients, they must paid £10 per day for the first ten days of public in-patient care in any one year.

Category II and Category III were combined in legislation enacted in 1991 to produce a two-category system which is currently in existence.

All citizens are eligible for free care, including in-patient care, for communicable diseases and certain chronic diseases, and for infant screening and child health examinations.

Turning to insurance cover, about 30 % of the population had health insurance policies with the Voluntary Health Insurance Board in 1987. The Board offers two main types of policy: broad policies which cover private specialist fees, private or semi-private hospital accommodation, and certain out-patient costs such as GPs' fees over a certain threshold; and narrow policies which cover only gaps in eligibility such as charges for public beds and hospital specialists' services. The great bulk of subscribers carry the first type of policy and they include many Category II individuals who are entitled to fairly comprehensive free public care.

The combination of the three categories of eligibility and the presence or absence of insurance cover meant that before recent reforms, there were at least six patient groups (see Table 6.2). During a typical episode of acute care, each group could face different financial incentives. Moreover, the methods by which doctors were paid

Table 6.1. **Eligibility for free health services and health insurance cover, 1987**

	Without Insurance (% population)	With Insurance	Total
Category I	36	1	37
Category II	32	16	48
Category III	4	11	15
Total	72	28	100

Source: Estimated from Commission on Health Funding (1989), and Nolan, 1991.

Table 6.2. **Access to health care: eligibility and insurance coverage, 1989**

	Eligibility for free (public) health services	Examples of additional cover with health insurance policies from the VHI
Category I:	1. Public in-patient care 2. Specialist doctor services 3. Maternity and infant welfare services 4. All prescribed medicines 5. Dental, ophthalmic and aural services 6. General practitioner care 7. All other publicly funded health services	E.g. *add* semi-private accommodation in public hospitals, plus treatment in private hospitals and private specialist doctor's fees.
Category II:	1. Public in-patient care subject to a £10 charge per day for the first 10 days in any one year 2. Specialist doctor services subject to a £10 charge for the first visit for any one condition 3. Maternity and infant welfare services 4. Prescribed medicines after the first £28 per month, or in the case of certain chronic illnesses 5. All other publicly funded health services (excluding 5 and 6 in Category I above)	E.g. *add* private accommodation in public hospitals, plus treatment in private hospitals, private specialist doctor's fees and GP and out-patient expenses, excluding the first £170 per year for a family (£100 for an individual) subject to a £1 200 ceiling.
Category III:	1. Public in-patent care subject to a £10 charge per day for the first 10 days in any one year 4. Prescribed medicines after the first £28 per month, or in case of certain chronic illnesses 5. All other publicly funded health services (excluding 2, 3, 5 and 6 under Category I above)	E.g. *add* private accommodation in public hospitals plus treatment and medical extras in private hospitals, private specialist doctors' fees, and GP and out-patient expenses, excluding the first £170 per year for a family (£100 for an individual) subject to a £1 400 ceiling.

Note: Category III was merged into Category II in 1991.

varied between some of the groups. Table 6.1 provides estimates of the numbers in each eligibility category and of those with or without insurance cover.

RELATIONSHIP BETWEEN THE POPULATION AND THIRD-PARTY PAYERS

Ireland has fewer third-party health service funders than most OECD countries. There are only two of any importance: the Department of Health (or central government) and the Voluntary Health Insurance Board (VHI). In 1987, central government accounted for about 78 % of total health expenditure, the VHI for about 9 %, leaving about 13 % for direct payments (Stationery Office, 1989, Table 4.1).

Central government expenditure is raised mainly from general taxation; there is also a specific health contribution levied at the rate of 1.25 % on the income of non-medical card holders, up to a ceiling of £15 500 in the 1988/89 tax year. However, this accounts for only about 5 % of total health expenditure. The Department of Finance has the capacity to exert tight central control over the level of public expenditure on health in each budget period.

The Voluntary Health Insurance Board is unusual in that it is sponsored and directly regulated by central government, yet offers voluntary insurance. The Board was designed to provide a complement to tax-funded health services which concentrate on the less well-off (McDowell, 1989). It has a monopoly of voluntary health insurance which has enabled it to adopt community rating from the outset and, more recently, to exert monopsony power over providers. A fairly limited range of seven main policies are available (for details see Commission on Health Funding, 1989). Like most private insurance, cover is excluded for existing medical conditions for new subscribers and there is an upper age limit at 64 for entry. Membership of the VHI grew rapidly in the late 1970s and early 1980s before levelling off at about 30 % of the population in the mid-1980s. The VHI used to provide most of its benefits in the form of reimbursement of medical care bills. In recent years, however, it has switched to paying specialists and hospitals directly.

Health insurance premiums are eligible for income-tax relief at subscriber's marginal rate of tax which ranged from a standard rate of 35 % to a top rate of 58 % in the 1988/89 tax year (OECD, 1989). In addition, income-tax relief is available for certain unreimbursed medical expenses exceeding £50 in one year for an individual or £100 a year for a family. Expenditure on routine maternity, dental and ophthalmic care is excluded from tax relief. In 1988, tax expenditures accounted for 3 % of health expenditure.

RELATIONSHIP BETWEEN THE THIRD-PARTY PAYERS AND THE PROVIDERS

Until 1989, most GPs were paid on a fee-for-service basis for Category I patients. Fees have then been replaced by capitation payments, weighted by age, sex and distance from patient, supplemented by fees for a few, specified procedures. There are no practice allowances (akin to salary payments) in GPs' remuneration, unlike the payment system in the United Kingdom. A few GPs continue to be paid by salary. About 1 500 of Ireland's 1 800 GPs take part in the public scheme for Category I patients. Normally, there is a limit of 2 000 on a doctor's list of medical card holders. Doctors usually have discretion over whether or not they accept patients onto their lists, but, under certain circumstances, they may be assigned patients by the GMS (Payments) Board. Another 48 % of the female population is eligible for free maternity care, and participating GPs are paid by fee for service for such care. Fees and capitation payments are negotiated between representatives of the doctors and the Department of Health. The fees per item paid by the GMS (Payments) Board were about 60 % of those prevailing for private patients in 1987.

Broadly speaking, health authorities pay chemists' dispensing fees and the ingredient costs of prescribed drugs which are supplied free of charge to eligible patients. However, the rates of payment differ according to whether the patient has Category I status or is eligible under the scheme for chronically ill patients in Categories II or III. Category II or III patients who incur pharmaceutical expenses in excess of £28 in a month can obtain refunds from the Health Board for amounts over £28. A limited list of drugs can be prescribed for eligible patients: the exclusions mainly concern medicines which can be bought over the counter. Drug prices are controlled under an agreement with the pharmaceutical industry which links prices to those in the United Kingdom. This provides control of retail prices for private patients because there is a standard chemists' mark-up of 50 % on the wholesale price of the drug.

Public general, special and long-stay hospitals receive annual, global budgets for operating costs which are not covered by fee-paying patients. Typically, there are increments each year for inflation, changes in service provision and government policy on the rate of growth of expenditure. Voluntary general hospitals receive their budgets direct from the Department of Health. Other public hospitals receive their budgets from the health boards which themselves receive budgets from the Department. The process of setting budgets has been mainly "top down" in recent years: that is to say it has been determined mainly by the Department of Health. However, there is an element of negotiation, involving an assessment of hospitals' needs, prior to the setting of budgets. An element of bidding or negotiation is also involved in the allocation of supplementary funds made available for particular service initiatives, such as tackling waiting times. Detailed analysis of alternative methods of allocating resources, including the application of case-mix based approaches, has been undertaken and is continuing. There is no accounting for depreciation of the capital stock or for interest. Major capital expenditure is financed by capital grants and is under the direct control of the Department of Health.

Private hospitals rely heavily on payments by private patients who carry insurance with the VHI. The VHI tries to indemnify its members for the full cost of the specific hospital accommodation covered under its policies. It has used its monopsony power to bargain on fees with the private hospitals. On occasions, the Board has opposed the opening of new private hospitals and has tried to persuade private hospitals to make more use of day care and to reduce the average length of stay (Voluntary Health Insurance Board, 1987). It now pays public and private hospitals directly for services provided to its members.

Before 1991, only Category I and II patients were entitled to free or heavily subsidised care as out-patients or in-patients by medical specialists. Since Category III was merged with Category II in 1991, this has applied to all residents. About 40 % of specialists are consultants who can take full responsibility for patients and are allowed to have private patients. The rest are junior doctors who work mainly in public hospitals. About 90 % of consultants have appointments in public hospitals and the vast majority of these have "full-time" contracts. A new contract was agreed with the hospital consultants in 1991, under which consultants could commit to different categories of hospital appointments. These appointments varied in salary levels and the facility to work in private practice, in association with the service commitment in public hospital. Consultants are paid by salary for their work with public patients, as are junior doctors. They are paid by fee for service for private patients, including, until 1991, all those with Category III eligibility.

GOVERNMENT PLANNING AND REGULATION

The public sector plays a dominant role in financing and, to a lesser extent, in providing and managing health care. About four-fifths of total health expenditure in the late 1980s was public, and another 9 % passed through the VHI, which, in some respects, acts as a public body. On the providing side, 74 % of beds are in public hospitals and most of the community health services are provided by the eight health boards.

This has enabled central government to exert considerable control, directly or indirectly, over the rate of growth of health expenditure and over the shape and pattern of health services. Ireland is one of those few OECD countries which has succeeded not just in reducing the rate of growth of public expenditure on health but in making absolute cuts in real expenditure during the 1980s. Relatively small areas of the health sector – mainly private GP services – are left to be shaped by market forces.

In addition to the various public financing and management mechanisms discussed above, the government exerts some control over numbers of doctors through limits applied by the education authorities on the places available for medical students, and through a committee (*Comhairle na nOspideal*) which regulates the number and type of consultant medical staff in hospitals and advises the Minister of Health on the organisation and operation of hospital services. Although central government makes few attempts to influence the clinical activities of doctors, the GMS (Payments) Board scrutinises the activity and prescribing of GPs who provide services for medical card holders, and investigates those claims which are significantly higher than average.

RECENT REFORMS

In 1989, the government introduced capitation payments in place of fee-for-service payments for the care provided to medical card holders (Category I patients) by most general practitioners. This was the most important reform of the past decade prior to the Report of the Commission on Health Funding. It was introduced because of concerns that the fee-for-service method of paying GPs (the level of fee was about 60 % of that for private patients) encouraged over-visiting, over-prescribing and the medicalisation of minor illnesses (Commission on Health Funding, 1989). Indeed, there was some evidence of higher consultation rates, especially return visits, by medical card holders, and of higher prescribing levels for these patients.

The new method of paying GPs introduces capitation payments weighted by the age of the patient (in five bands), the sex of the patient, and the distance between the patient's home and the doctor's practice (in 20 categories depending on the five age bands and four distance bands). In addition, there are extra out-of-hours payments and special payments for a few items of service. The scheme allows for superannuation and various forms of leave payments (for details, see Commission on Health Funding, 1989, Appendix 11A).

A series of other reforms were introduced since the end of the 1970s:

- In 1979, Category III patients were granted eligibility for free care in public beds but they remained responsible for consultants' fees;
- Between 1981 and 1983, a new consultants' contract was negotiated, placing all consultants on salary for their services to public patients. Previously, consultants in voluntary hospitals had been paid by a mixture of sessional payments for out-patients and per-patient-day payments for in-patients;
- In 1982, about 900 items, mainly over the counter medicines, were removed from the list of drugs which could be prescribed under the public scheme;
- In 1983, manufacturers' drug prices were tied to those in the United Kingdom;
- In 1983 and in 1984, the threshold for patients to claim back pharmaceutical expenditure under the drugs subsidy scheme was raised;

- Charges for private and semi-private accommodation in public hospitals were increased substantially in real terms on several occasions;
- In 1987, £10 charges for first out-patient visits and for the first 10 days of in-patient care in public beds were introduced for Category II patients, and Category III patients became liable for the in-patient charges if they used a public bed. These charges were increased to £12.50 in 1991.
- In 1991, Category III was merged into Category II following a recommendation of the Commission on Health Funding.

GROWTH AND PERFORMANCE

The Irish health care system combines public and voluntary finance with public and private provision. The most important source of finance is general taxation, and central government has considerable discretion over the rate of growth of expenditure. That such discretion exists is illustrated by the rate of growth of health expenditure in the 1980s.

The economy went through a difficult period between 1980 and 1986; in four of the six years there was negative economic growth (OECD, 1989). The government responded by restraining sharply the growth of nominal public expenditure in the light of evidence which suggested that Ireland enjoyed comparatively high levels of public spending compared with countries with a similar standard of living. Public expenditure on health services actually fell in real terms in most of the years between 1980 and 1990 and by the end of this period it was down 8 % in real terms. This was accompanied by a 29 % decline in the number of acute hospital beds, a 29 % decline in average length of stay and a 13 % fall in admission rates.

According to OECD figures, there was a compensating rise in real private expenditure, by 55 %, and the private share of total spending rose from about 18 % to about 21 % in 1990. However, since private expenditure was much smaller than public expenditure, total real health expenditure still fell by 5 % over the period (Poullier, 1989). VHI premiums rose by 46 % in real terms between 1980 and 1988 (Commission on Health Funding, 1989). Although this rise was steep, it was lower than the real rise of 91 % in the average claim per person covered under private health insurance in the United Kingdom over the same period. Although this comparison is blurred by changes in membership and policies in both markets, it is tempting to conclude that the difference between the two figures reflects differences in the structure of the two insurance industries: regulated monopsony in Ireland and unregulated competition in Great Britain. The rise in premiums in Ireland was backed by an extraordinary surge of 350 % in tax relief over the period, taking it to about 28 % of VHI premiums on average (Commission on Health Funding, 1989, Table 4.3, deflated by figures in Poullier, 1989, Table 13).

The decline in total health expenditure showed up, also, as a fall in the share of GDP devoted to health, from 9.2 % in 1980 to 7.0 % in 1990. This is the sharpest fall (24 %) recorded among OECD countries over this period (see Chapter 10). To some extent, this can be seen as a reaction to the unusually rapid growth in the share of GDP devoted to health in the 1970s – from 5.6 % in 1970 to 9.2 % in 1980.

Health expenditure per head was US$ 607 in 1987, 21 % higher than that in Spain, 81 % of that in the United Kingdom and 27 % of that in the United States. This was somewhat above the level which would be expected on the basis of a regression line linking GDP per capita to health expenditure per capita among major OECD countries (Schieber and Poullier, 1989).

According to OECD (1987), Schieber *et al.* (1991) and Table 10.2, Ireland had fairly typical rates per capita of prescriptions, acute hospital beds, and acute hospital admissions in the early 1980s. However, it had: an unusually low average length of in-patient stay in acute hospitals (7.4 days in 1986); one of the lowest levels of doctors per 1 000 (1.5 in 1987 compared with an average of 2.5 among the seven countries in this book) and a low level of physician contacts per capita (4.0 in 1980 judging by data obtained by Tussing, 1985). The low level of physician contacts is likely to have been mainly the result of the exposure of about 30 % of the population to all fees for GP care and another 30 % of the population to fees costing less than £ 100 in a year for an individual. Data on waiting times for hospital admission are not published routinely but a survey suggested that, in 1980, 7.8 % of all in-patients waited more than one month for admission to hospital and 1.6 % waited for more than one year (Tussing, 1985).

Turning to health status, in 1986, expectation of life at birth was 77 years for females and 71 years for males. Perinatal mortality was 0.99 % in 1989 (Table 10.3). The life expectancy rates are towards the bottom end of the range for OECD countries and the perinatal mortality figure towards the top end of the range. Although it is difficult to be precise about what exactly determines health status in any country, these figures are as likely to have resulted from relatively modest standard of living as from the performance of the health services. Perinatal mortality has declined steadily in the past three decades and it continued to decline between 1980 and 1989, despite only modest economic growth through 1987 and real cuts in health expenditure.

Turning to the question of access to acute health care, the combination of eligibility categories and the availability of private health insurance means that different groups of patients face different financial incentives (see Tables 6.1 and 6.2). And depending on whether the patients are public or private, the providers are also presented with different incentives. Occasional household surveys have explored the effects of consumer and provider incentives on the way in which health care is used.

Tussing (1985) carried out a household survey in 1980 which included questions on medical care utilisation, age, sex, occupation, eligibility category and insurance cover, but not health status. He used regression analysis to explore the determinants of utilisation. His tests of three hypotheses are worth reporting:

Hypothesis I: That since Category I patients received free care from GPs paid by fee for service, they would have more visits, and more return visits for any initial visit, than Category II or III patients who were obliged to pay for their care. This was borne out strongly both by the crude data, which showed that Category I patients had 2.5 times as many visits as Category II and Category III patients, and by regression analysis which controlled for some of the potentially confounding variables. It was likely that the poor health status of Category I patients played a part in this result. However, comparisons between Irish and British GP consultation rates suggested that whereas the lower occupational groups had higher consultation rates than the higher occupational groups in *both* countries, the lower occupational groups had *relatively* much higher rates in Ireland. Since all British groups enjoy free GP care and British GPs are paid mainly by capitation and salary, this suggested that the restriction of free care to the lower occupational groups in Ireland, combined with fee-for-service payment of GPs, played a part in raising consultation rates by Category I patients independently of health status.

Hypothesis II: That fee-for-service payment of GPs for Category I patients would encourage doctors to induce demand by asking such patients to make return visits. More specifically, return visits would be higher when doctors' incomes came under pressure, such as when the doctor/population ratio was higher, other things being equal. The analysis established that return visits were, indeed, higher the greater the doctor/ population ratio. Since Tussing completed his analysis, further evidence has emerged suggestive of GP-induced demand associated with pressure on their incomes. Visiting rates for Category I patients rose by 12 %, from 5.8 per capita in 1980 to 6.5 per capita in 1987 at a time when rises in fees for Category I patients were declining by about 10 % in real terms. There was no evidence of rising consultation rates for other categories of patient judging by the available household surveys (Commission on Health Funding, 1989, page 209). Such divergent trends are reminiscent of comparisons between physician payment systems in Canada and the United States (Barer, Evans and Labelle, 1988).

Hypothesis III: That Category II and III patients with VHI cover would make more visits to GPs than patients without such cover. This was borne out by the analysis but it remained unclear whether the effect was due to health status and to adverse selection rather than to moral hazard.

Nolan (1991) was able to explore some of these relationships more thoroughly using a 1987 household survey which included data on health status and income in addition to data on the household characteristics included in Tussing's survey. The health status variable was a simple dichotomy between those suffering from a serious illness or disability and those who were not. The survey took place at a time when GPs were still being paid by fee for service for Category I patients. Nolan found crude differences in visiting rates between Category I patients and other patients, similar to those found by Tussing. He showed that, other things being equal, health status was indeed an important determinant of these differences. However, whereas the inclusion of the health status variable in regression analysis similar to that carried out by Tussing reduced the explanatory power of Category I eligibility over the total number of GP visits in the year, it by no means removed it altogether.

Although the crudeness of the health status variable could have accounted for these results, the suggestion remains that patient and doctor incentives play an independent part in determining utilisation of GP services. Nolan also showed that health insurance cover was associated positively and significantly with visits to GPs and with hospital utilisation and length of stay, after allowing for other explanatory variables, including health status. However, given the simple nature of the health status variable used, the effect of health insurance might have been over-estimated.

Further evidence on the effect of provider incentives on activity rates was forthcoming in the wake of the switch, in March 1989, from fee-for-service to capitation payments for GPs providing care to Category I patients. Early reports suggested that consultation rates fell by about 20 % in the first year.

Publicly provided services

A distinctive mixture of public and private health care finance and provision has given the entire Irish population access to comprehensive services which are of high quality. Furthermore, the cost of supplying public services has been distributed across the entire population according to a taxation regime which is slightly progressive (Rottman and Reidy, 1988). The eligibility system entirely protects lower income groups from the hardship which would be associated with paying medical bills. All this has been achieved in a system in which expenditure on health, although it grew very rapidly in the 1970s, was cut back sharply during the 1980s.

However, there are persistent weaknesses in the Irish system, similar to those being experienced in other OECD countries. The period of rapid growth in expenditure (especially public expenditure) illustrated the tendency for health care systems which are financed largely by third parties to grow at unacceptably high rates unless checked. When a third party, such as the government, is paying for most health care, the patient has no incentive to economise. When, as in the Irish system before 1989, the GP, who acts as a gatekeeper, is paid by fee for service for public patients there are positive incentives for such doctors to induce demand.

The government was successful during the 1980s in countering the underlying tendencies in the system towards excessive public expenditure. It used methods such as control of GPs' fees (but not volume), tightening of global, block budgets in public hospitals, reducing beds, closing hospitals and greater reliance on salary payments for hospital specialists. At the end of the decade, there was a switch to capitation payments for the public patients of GPs. However, these measures were accompanied by a slight drop in public hospital admission rates, reports of lengthening waiting lists and strong protests about deteriorating access for public patients. These well-tried and effective systems for capping the expenditure of the providers also brought with them certain well-known, if potential, problems for incentives.

In the case of GPs, there is a risk that capitation payments will lead to underservice in place of overservice. This can be avoided if patients are in a position to identify poorly performing GPs and to change to another doctor. In other words, competition can be a safeguard against underservice. In the case of hospitals, tight block budgets are not designed to reward good performance. Competition between public hospitals has not yet been encouraged in Ireland. Hospital consultants who are salaried may be tempted to underserve their patients, especially when there is competition for their time from fee-paying patients. There is also the possibility that they may delegate work inappropriately to junior doctors. All this may generate failures in responsiveness to patients.

Some commentators have also been critical of the way in which the publicly provided health services are managed, and of weaknesses in management information. In particular, the Commission on Health Funding (1989) identified a confusion between political and executive functions; an inappropriate balance between national and local decision-making; insufficient involvement of clinicians in management; insufficient accountability; and insufficient integration of related services. The Commission also pointed to severe gaps in information, particularly on the costs of treatment, the need for services, and the outcome and quality of care.

Privately financed services

There are few causes for concern about the few health services where the patient pays the provider out-of-pocket for the full cost of care. The system has been designed so that it is mainly those who can afford to pay, and who choose not to have insurance, who are left in this situation. Their choices and those of their doctors are made in full awareness of the costs, although tax relief is available after a certain point on unreimbursed medical expenses. In practice, however, claims for such tax relief are few in number.

However, 30 % of the population is now covered by private health insurance with the VHI which has a monopoly of such insurance. There are three concerns here: risk selection, moral hazard, and tax relief.

   i) The VHI has used its monopoly power to establish community rating. This policy is popular because it favours those individuals with relatively poor health. However, it has almost certainly encouraged adverse selection of VHI policies by high-risk individuals (Nolan, 1991) and relative underconsumption of such policies by the healthy.
   ii) Most policies cover the full cost of a specified type of in-patient care and the cost of all GP and out-patient care after the first £100 for an individual and the first £170 for a family. This means that privately insured patients face no financial incentives to economise after the out-patient deductible is exceeded. Their doctors are invariably paid by fee for service which provides them with positive

incentives to induce demand. It is not surprising, therefore, that VHI premiums rose by 46 % in real terms between 1980 and 1988.

In the late 1980s, the government constrained the rate of increase of premiums of the VHI. This, combined with a policy of unrestrained, cost-based reimbursement for hospital bills, led to a financial crisis in 1989 because claims grew faster than premiums. Measures had to be taken to reduce members' entitlements, to negotiate global financial agreements with private hospitals and to agree tighter definitions within fee schedules with the medical profession.

iii) Tax relief accounted for about 28 % of the cost of VHI premiums in 1987, having risen by 350 % in real terms since 1980. There are a number of problems with granting tax relief for private health insurance, particularly at the marginal rate of income tax. It is inequitable because it favours those on higher incomes more than those on lower incomes. It is inefficient because it lowers the price of insurance, thereby encouraging individuals to take out cover they would not otherwise buy. This reduces awareness of the cost of premium rises and, given the moral hazard associated with health insurance, is akin to pouring petrol on a fire. Compared with direct public expenditure on health services, tax relief is poorly targeted on medical need. It can be used to pay for treatments and hotel luxuries, which would not be provided under a public scheme, and for priority access to doctors by private patients.

Frontiers between the public and the private sectors

Many of the weaknesses in the way the system works may be seen most clearly as strains and stresses on the frontiers between the public and private health sectors, particularly in public hospitals. The Commission on Health Funding received ample testimony that private patients in public hospitals enjoyed shorter waiting times and more personal attention from consultants than public patients. It also heard suggestions that some consultants were not fulfilling the terms of their public contracts. There have been reports (Lancet, 1989) that the cuts in public expenditure and the growth of private practice have led to lengthening waiting lists and premature discharge of public patients, not forgetting the sharp drop in hospital admissions in recent years.

There are sound economic and policy reasons for allowing private care in public hospitals. It can help to give public as well as private patients access to the best doctors and it can provide a welcome source of revenue for the public sector. However, there are likely to be equity difficulties within the public sector if public and private care are not kept financially separate. Two important principles are that there should be a clear financial separation between public and private transactions and that the private patient should pay the full cost of the service that he or she receives. Otherwise, there is a danger that public funds and resources will be diverted according to private preferences and ability to pay.

In Ireland, the main problem seems to be the extent to which there are subsidies to private care. The extent of which was noted in relation to private insurance. Furthermore, there was an anomaly in that Category III patients were allowed to use a public bed while enjoying the private services of a consultant. This is no longer the case following the 1991 legislation. In addition, there were also subsidies built into the pricing of private and semi-private beds in public hospitals, although these seem to have been virtually phased out by sharp increases in private bed charges in the 1980s.

COMMISSION ON HEALTH FUNDING

The sharp cuts in real public expenditure on health were largely responsible for the financing and organisation of health care becoming politically controversial during the 1980s. The government responded by appointing the Commission on Health Funding in June 1987 with terms of reference, "To examine the financing of the health services and to make recommendations on the extent and sources of the future funding required to provide an equitable, comprehensive and cost-effective public health service and on any changes in administration which seem desirable for that purpose".

The Commission reported in September 1989 with an evaluation of health services which, in many ways – and despite some fairly radical proposals for reform – represented a vote of confidence in the health care system. The Commission's main conclusions and recommendations are considered hereafter.

Financing, eligibility and the public/private mix

The level of health funding could only be decided according to the available resources and the priority attached by society to different social objectives. It noted that allocative decisions in the health care field were often based on intuitive rather than objective criteria. On equity, it concluded essentially in favour of payment according to means, and access to services in relation to medical need.

Having explored various alternative funding mechanisms, it came down in favour of continuing reliance mainly on public funding, with private finance playing a supplementary role. The majority of the Commission's members favoured continuing dependence on general taxation but there was a minority report in favour of an earmarked health tax. The small, existing health contribution element of taxation should, however, be abolished.

Although the Commission favoured public *funding* of services, it declared that it made no presumption in favour of public *provision*. On the contrary, there should be flexibility for the public authorities in each area to turn to private providers (or to public providers in other areas) if this would be more cost-effective than direct provision. The Commission gave some cautious endorsement to the advantages of competition and competitive tendering among hospitals, nursing homes and domiciliary providers. However, it envisaged competitive tendering for the management of hospitals rather than changes in contracts which would affect the availability of facilities themselves.

On the three levels of eligibility for free public care, the Commission recommended, essentially, that there be no change to Categories I and II and abolition of Category III. This meant that the lowest income group would still be eligible for all health services, free of charge. The rest of the population would be entitled to core services free of charge, covering: all hospital care (subject to existing charges); a range of health services in the community, excluding GP services; and prescribed drugs costing more than £28 per month and for people suffering from certain chronic diseases. It also meant that patients would have to choose between public and private in-patient care. They would not be able to combine a public bed with a private consultant's services.

The Commission rejected any significant increase in user charges for public services, while accepting the principle of modest direct contributions. It envisaged continuation of private care and private health insurance. Consequential inequities in access would be acceptable provided adequate standards of public care were preserved. While it expressed support for community rating, it hesitated over the future of the VHI monopoly, partly because of doubts about its efficiency, but mainly because of uncertainty as to whether it could continue after the completion of the internal market of the European Community.

The Commission recommended the phasing out of tax relief for private health insurance on the grounds that this was inequitable and poorly targeted on need. Its recommendation about universal access to core services free of charge further undermined the case for tax relief.

Administration, management and management information

The kernel of the Commission's conclusions was that the solution to the financing question did not lie primarily in the system of funding, but rather in the way that services were planned, organised and delivered. In this connection, the Commission made a number of recommendations:

- The Minister's policy and management roles should be separated and the latter should be transferred to an executive authority with a chief executive and area general managers at the level of the existing health boards;
- The health boards should be transformed into health councils charged with playing a local policy role, representing consumer interests and monitoring the quality of care;
- There should be clarification of the role of voluntary hospitals and agencies and they should be funded for an agreed level and type of service;
- There should be a performance audit unit.

The Commission also laid stress on the need for better management information and evaluation. A number of recommendations were made for health population profiles, better measurement of effectiveness, and better measurement of costs. There should be more cost-benefit analysis and more health technology assessment. The Health Executive should acquire the services of qualified and experienced clinicians to assist in performance evaluation. Epidemiological and health services research should be strengthened.

The services

The Commission recommended that all public hospitals should be given clear objectives and should be funded according to an agreed level of services based on activities and unit costs classified by diagnosis-related groups (DRG). An important step in this direction was the completion of a major study developing DRGs for acute in-patients in Ireland and the piloting of a DRG costing procedure in three acute hospitals (Wiley and Fetter, 1990).

There should be common waiting lists for public and private patients in public hospitals and publication of maximum waiting times. In addition, there should be monitoring of the public time commitment of consultants.

The linking of drug prices to those in the United Kingdom should be terminated in favour of a limited list of drugs for which prices would be negotiated directly with the drug companies.

Measures should be taken to strengthen prevention and health promotion.

There should be better evaluation of alternatives for long-term care and better co-ordination of the existing services.

PROPOSALS EVALUATED

There are parallels between the Commission's proposals and the current reforms to the health care system in the United Kingdom – for example, tighter management in the public sector, competition among providers, better representation for consumers and improved management information. The Commission, however, was cautious in its endorsement of competition among providers. The proposals for making free access to core services available to all Irish citizens, reducing the tiers of eligibility to two and phasing out tax relief, seem well judged when viewed against the objective of improving the balance between public and private patients, particularly in public hospitals.

The Commission was ambivalent in its support for the VHI, although it favoured continuation of community rating. It may have underestimated the advantages which a regulated, monopsony insurer has over competitive insurers in holding down the rate of increase of private sector costs, as well as insurance premiums. Given the competition policy of the European Community, however, it is not clear that the option of allowing the monopsony to continue is available.

The Commission's report was followed in 1990 by the report of the Stationery Office. The Review Body's main recommendations on the remuneration and terms and conditions of employment of consultant medical staff included:

- The introduction of new categories of consultant posts and mechanisms which would entail higher remuneration for greater commitment by consultants to the public sector;
- Clearer definitions of the responsibilities of consultants and of the hospitals in which they worked;
- More involvement of clinicians in management;
- The introduction of contractual arrangements to support the introduction of medical audit systems, and
- Significant increases in consultants' remuneration.

WAY FORWARD

The government's response to the findings of the Commission on Health Funding was to welcome the overall thrust of the report, while making no immediate decisions on either structural reform or funding arrangements. During 1991, however, legislation was introduced to merge eligibility Category III into Category II, resulting in a two-tier eligibility system. The government also accepted the recommendations of the Review Body on the remuneration and terms and conditions of employment of consultant medical staff as a basis for further discussions with the medical profession. In 1991, a national agreement between all the social partners (government, employers, trade unions, farmers) included a commitment to the establishment of a Performance Audit Unit in Department of House (Stationery Office, 1991a). In 1990, the Minister for Health announced an "action plan" for the health services with the aim of improving their efficiency and effectiveness. The Dublin Hospital Initiative Group which participated in this strategy reported in 1991, and recommended the establishment of a Regional Hospital Authority in Dublin, outside of the Health Board Structure. This, and other proposals, for structural reform are currently being considered (Stationery Office, 1991b). These reforms are likely to reduce some of the ambiguities and tensions on the boundaries between public and private health care. They are also likely to contribute to better management, both in hospitals and in ambulatory care.

References

Barer, M. L., Evans, R. G. and Labelle, R. J. (1988), "Fee Controls as Cost Control: Tales from the Frozen North", *The Milbank Quarterly,* Vol. 66, No. 1.

Hensey, B. (1988), *The Health Services of Ireland,* Institute of Public Administration, Dublin.

The Lancet (1989), "Irish Electorate Speaks on Health", July 8.

McCarthy, D. (1984), "Principles for the Allocation of Resources in Health Care", *Future Directions in Health Policy,* pp. 13-37, Paper of a Conference held in Malahide, Co., Dublin, 6-7 April.

McDowell, M. (1989), "Examination of the Report of the Commission on Health Funding", typescript, University College, Dublin, 6 November.

Nolan, B. (1991), "Health Services Utilisation and Financing in Ireland", The Economic and Social Research Institute, General Research Series Paper No. 155, Dublin.

OECD (1987), *Financing and Delivering Health Care,* Paris.

OECD (1989), *OECD Economic Surveys: Ireland 1988/1989,* Paris.

Poullier, J. P. (1990), "Compendium, Health Care Expenditure and other Data", in *Health Systems in Transition,* OECD.

Raftery, J. (1984), "Irish Health Service Expenditure: Policy Trends and Incentives", *Future Directions in Health Policy,* pp. 77-94, Papers of a Conference held in Malahide, Co., Dublin, 6-7 April.

Raftery, J. (1988), "Lessons from the Irish", *The Health Service Journal,* pp. 1064-65, 15 September.

Rottman, D. and Reidy, M. (1988), *Redistributive Effect of State Transfer Payments,* National Economic and Social Council, Dublin.

Schieber, G. J. and Poullier, J. P. (1989), "International Health Care Expenditure Trends: 1987", *Health Affairs,* Fall, pp. 169-177.

Schieber, G.J., Poullier, J. P. and Greenwald, L. M., (1991), "Health Care Systems in Twenty-Four Countries", *Health Affairs,* Fall.

Sláinte, An Roinn (1986), *Health: The Wider Dimensions (A Consultative Statement on Health Policy),* Department of Health, Dublin, November.

Stationery Office (1989), *Report of the Commission on Health Funding,* Dublin, September.

Stationery Office (1990), *Report of the Review Body on Higher Remuneration in the Public Sector: Hospital Consultants,* Dublin.

Stationery Office (1991*a*), *Programme for Economic and Social Progress,* Dublin.

Stationery Office (1991*b*), *Report of the Dublin Hospital Initiative Group,* Dublin.

Tussing, A. D. (1985), *Irish Medical Care Resources: An Economic Analysis,* The Economic and Social Research Institute, Dublin, Paper 126, November.

Voluntary Health Insurance Board (1987), *30th Annual Report and Accounts for year ending 28th February 1987,* Dublin.

Wiley, M. M. and Fetter, R. B. (1990), *Measuring Activity and Costs in Irish Hospitals: a Study of Hospital Case-Mix,* The Economic and Social Research Institute, Dublin.

Chapter 7

THE REFORM OF THE HEALTH SYSTEM IN THE NETHERLANDS

INTRODUCTION

In 1986, the then centre-right Dutch government appointed a committee chaired by Dr. W. Dekker to advise on strategies for reforming the structure and financing of the health care system in the Netherlands. The Dekker Committee reported in March 1987, following which the government proposed major structural changes to the health care system (Ministry of Welfare, Health and Cultural Affairs 1988). Following a change of government in November 1989, the new centre-left administration decided to continue with the main thrust of the reforms. What is proposed is probably the most radical health care reform so far planned for the 1990s in any OECD country:

- A uniform scheme of national health insurance (or "basic" insurance) for all residents in the Netherlands;
- Integration of both health care and related social services under the scheme; and
- A decisive movement away from direct government involvement in the determination of the volume and price of health services towards regulated competition, both in the market for health insurance and in the market for health care itself.

This chapter describes those reforms and assesses some likely benefits and difficulties which may arise once they are introduced. We begin by describing the existing health care system – including its growth and performance – and go on to discuss the problems which gave rise to the need for reforms.

THE HEALTH CARE SYSTEM BEFORE THE REFORMS

Health care in the Netherlands is supplied mainly by independent practitioners and by private, non-profit institutions, although there are some public hospitals. The system is financed by a mixture of social and private insurance contributions combined with significant direct payments and government subsidies. The whole population is compulsorily insured for chronic health care risks. A little over 30% of the population relies on voluntary insurance for acute health care risks. The remaining 70% is compulsorily insured for acute health care risks. The system represents a mixture of the voluntary reimbursement model and the public contract model, outlined in Chapter 2. Tight and detailed central regulation of prices, volume and capacity has been superimposed on an essentially private system of provision and a mixed system of finance.

Chart 7.1 depicts some of the key relationships, financial and service in the system. At the bottom left of the diagram is the population, including patients. At the top centre are the insurers and third-party financing bodies. At the bottom right are the providers. Service flows are shown as solid lines, financing flows as broken lines. The diagram concentrates on core health services, neglecting, for example, dentistry and ophthalmic services. It excludes social services, such as homes for the elderly. Private insurers are shown as multiple because there is competition between them, but other insurers and providers are shown as single because competition between them is currently weak or non-existent. The diagram abstracts from many complications both in the insurance and in the provision sectors. It also abstracts from considerable government regulation of the quality, price and volume of care.

Chart 7.1 The health care system in the Netherlands in 1987

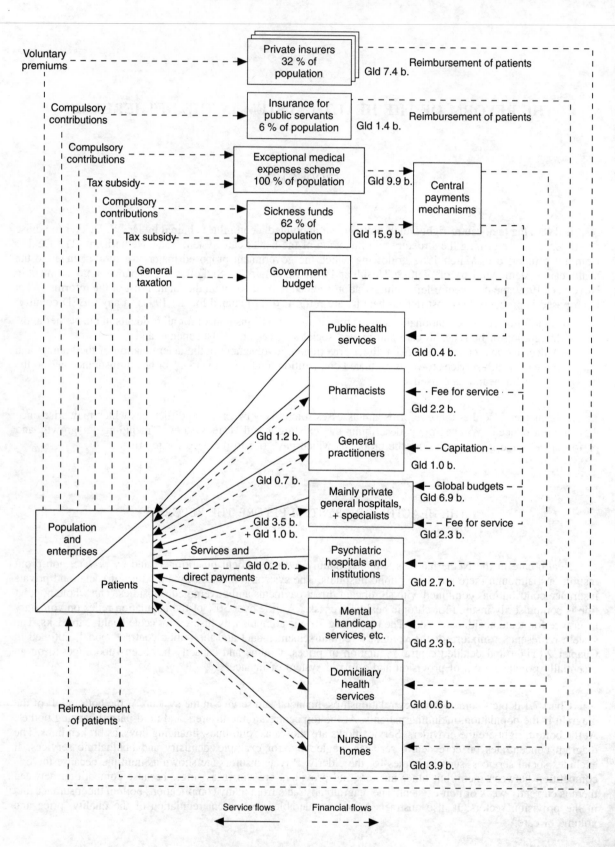

RELATIONSHIP BETWEEN PATIENTS AND PROVIDERS

Primary medical and pharmaceutical care

The general practitioner (GP) plays a key role because he or she provides nearly all primary medical care and acts as a gatekeeper for specialists and hospitals. GPs are independent contractors, with about one in two working in group practices or health centres. Some operate their own dispensaries; alternatively, the patient can take the GP's prescription to a pharmacist.

The sickness fund patient has to chose a GP with whom to register from among those with whom his/her sickness fund has a contract. In practice, the sickness funds have contracted with nearly all GPs in the region in which they work. The sickness fund pays the GP a capitation allowance and the GP provides free care to the patient. Privately insured patients and public employees are free to consult any GP however, and they pay by fee for service. They can claim back the fees from their insurer, provided they have not decided to bear the risk themselves.

Prescribed drugs are now provided free of charge to sickness fund patients, but private patients have to pay the pharmacist and claim reimbursement from their insurance company if drugs are included in their benefit package.

Specialist medical care

About one-third of medical consultations are with specialists. This compares with about one-quarter in the United Kingdom, but nearly one-half in Germany (Sandier, 1989). Specialists are usually associated with hospitals, but some have independent practices. Most specialists are paid for their service at fee levels which are controlled by the Central Agency for Health Care Tariffs. This applies to both private and sickness fund patients. Specialists in public and academic hospitals and junior doctors are salaried. Again, for sickness fund patients the bill is paid direct to the specialist by the sickness fund, but privately insured patients have to pay and claim back fees, depending on their insurance cover.

Hospitals and nursing homes

The Netherlands has about 12 health care beds per 1 000 population (OECD average about 9.3 in 1983). 42% are in general and specialist acute hospitals, 14% in psychiatric hospitals, 17% in institutions for the mentally handicapped and 27% in nursing homes. Only about 15% of acute hospitals are public. The rest are private, non-profit hospitals with their own independent governing bodies (Tiddens et al., 1984). There is some cost-sharing for long-term care facilities which accounts for about 10% of the costs.

Public health and domiciliary services

Public health services are managed by municipalities and financed out of taxation. Domiciliary health services are run mainly by the "Cross" organisations. These are financed by the exceptional medical expenses fund and, to a small extent, by direct payments by the clients.

RELATIONSHIP BETWEEN THE POPULATION AND THIRD-PARTY PAYERS

Sources of funds

In 1988 compulsory health insurance contributions accounted for about 60% of health expenditure. Subsidies out of general taxation accounted for about 14%, voluntary health insurance premiums for less than 16%, and out-of-pocket payments for about 11% of expenditure. The scale of voluntary premiums is slightly overstated, here, because of the inclusion of compulsory contributions by public servants who are treated as private patients.

Nearly all Dutch citizens have comprehensive health insurance cover. There are four main schemes:

- An exceptional medical expenses scheme covering the whole population;

- A compulsory (ordinary expenses) health insurance scheme covering mainly employees earning below a certain salary and corresponding retirees (about 60% of the population);
- Voluntary private insurance covering mainly employees earning above a certain salary and corresponding retirees (about 30% of the population);
- A compulsory health insurance scheme covering public employees and corresponding retirees (about 6% of the population).

A General Fund for Compulsory Insurance channels government contributions to the exceptional medical expenses scheme and to the sickness funds. There is also a separate programme for social care which covers the whole population.

Exceptional medical expenses scheme

This is a compulsory scheme for catastrophic health expenditure which covers the whole population. The scheme pays mainly for long-term care in nursing homes, in psychiatric institutions and in general hospitals when the duration of stay exceeds 365 days. It is financed mainly by income-related contributions (4.55% of earnings, up to a ceiling, in 1988) made by employees out of compulsory additions to wages by employers. The self-employed have to make their own contributions. There is a small tax subsidy and patients, or their relatives, may have to make a contribution to the cost of care. Providers are reimbursed directly for services provided in kind. The administration of benefits is handled by the individual's usual insurer. Negotiations with providers about individual beneficiaries are handled by a designated liaison fund (sickness fund) in each locality. Payments are made by a central payments office.

Sickness funds insurance

Since 1941, the Netherlands has had a compulsory health insurance scheme covering non-exceptional risks for employees earning below a certain income level. The current scheme has been widened, and now covers dependants, retirees from the scheme, and anybody receiving social security benefits provided they earn below a certain income limit (about Gld 50 000 in 1988). However, in 1986 membership was curtailed when the government abolished voluntary membership of sickness funds, requiring the self-employed and future retirees holding private insurance to take out or continue cover with private insurers. This reduced the percentage of the population covered by the sickness funds from 69 to 62%. Benefits under the compulsory scheme include GP and specialist care, maternity services, dental care, hospital services, pharmaceutical goods and transport services. Supplementary voluntary insurance is still available for compulsorily insured members to opt for higher standards of hospital accommodation.

The scheme is administered by about 40 independent, non-profit, sickness funds which are mainly geographically specialised. There is little competition between funds, as most have a monopoly position within the boundaries of its legally defined working area. To obtain benefits, individuals must register with a local sickness fund and with a general practitioner with whom the sickness fund has a contract. The scheme is financed mainly by income-related contributions for employees, until recently paid 50/50 by the employer and the employee. The contribution rate was 10.2% of earnings in 1988 up to a ceiling of about Gld 42 000. Contributions are collected by enterprises and sickness funds and are paid into a General Fund. There is also a tax subsidy. As mentioned above, sickness funds make contracts with providers (indeed, they are generally not allowed to refuse a contract) and make direct reimbursement for services supplied to their members. They undertake only limited utilisation reviews. They may also provide supplementary private insurance for extra services, such as higher classes of hospital care.

Private insurance

The self-employed and employees earning over a certain income limit, together with people over 65 formerly in these categories, can opt for cover for non-exceptional risks by one of 70 proprietary and non-profit private health insurers. Those who take out private insurance account for about 32% of the population. Private insurance is voluntary and individuals can carry some of the risk for themselves, but very few do not insure at all. Premiums are per individual and vary according to medical risk, the level of deductible chosen and the desired level of hospital accommodation (first, second or third class). Private insurance premiums are tax deductible only to the extent that they exceed an amount equal to an imputed compulsory contribution to a sickness fund on the income of the individual concerned. As mentioned above, private insurers usually indemnify the patient for fees paid to providers.

Traditionally, private insurance premiums were community-rated, but this arrangement began to break down in the 1970s. High-risk individuals, especially the elderly, were faced with steep rises in premiums. Rather than leaving the sickness funds to act as insurers of last resort, the government has obliged private insurers since 1989 to provide standard cover at set premiums, below cost, for people over 65 who were previously covered by private insurance. A system has been devised to spread the corresponding outgoings among other privately insured persons. In effect, this imposes social insurance conditions on private insurers (Ministry of Welfare, Health and Cultural Affairs, 1989).

Insurance for public employees

Public employees must join compulsory insurance schemes with benefits similar to those provided by sickness funds. Contributions are income-related and until recently have been shared 50/50 between employers and employees. Dependants and associated retirees are covered. Like private insurance, these schemes provide indemnity payments rather than benefits in kind. The schemes cover about 6% of the population.

The General Fund for Compulsory Insurance

The General Fund for Compulsory Insurance channels contributions to the exceptional medical expenses scheme and to the sickness funds. As well as acting as a central pool for contributions, it receives a government subsidy. Although the government sets contribution rates, payments by the Fund are potentially open-ended. Deficits or surpluses can be carried forward.

Social care

The whole population is eligible for social care, including domiciliary care and old people's homes. These services are financed by a mix of sources including the exceptional medical expenses fund, general taxation and out-of-pocket payments.

RELATIONSHIP BETWEEN THIRD-PARTY PAYERS AND PROVIDERS

Physicians

Although providers are generally paid directly by private patients, they are paid by public third parties for public patients. The sickness funds pay GPs by capitation for their members. They pay specialists for each patient referred to them by a GP. The patient is given a referral card which entitles him or her to treatment for one month. However, specialists are paid over and above this by fee for service for a long list of specific diagnostic and therapeutic procedures. The various fees and capitation allowances are negotiated in a complex way between representatives of the physicians and of the insurers with the involvement not only of the Central Agency on Health Care Tariffs but also the government. There are separate negotiations over the personal income of physicians and over payments for practice costs (Kirkman-Liff, 1989). There has been discussion about bringing in global budgets for payments to specialists which would have the effect of reducing automatically fees per item if the volume of services went up more than had been allowed for in the budget.

Pharmaceuticals

The pharmacist or dispensing doctor is reimbursed by the sickness fund for drugs prescribed to sickness fund members. There has been no control of the prices set by the manufacturers for pharmaceuticals, but the pharmacists' dispensing fee is set by negotiations between representatives of the insurers and the pharmacists and approved by the Central Agency for Health Care Tariffs. In July 1991, a list of reference prices for pharmaceutical ingredients has been introduced for the sickness funds and part of the private insurance market. The fixed refund price is based on the average list price for "therapeutically interchangeable" drugs (such as drugs within the Benzodiazepine group or the Insulin group). The manufacturer will remain free to charge higher prices and the doctor will remain free to prescribe a higher priced drug, but the patient will have to pay the difference.

Hospitals

Since 1983, hospitals have had prospective, annual, global budgets negotiated with local insurers, public and private, and approved by the Central Agency for Health Care Tariffs. Budgets cover both public and private patients and they cover most costs with the exception of fees for specialists. They replaced an earlier, volume-related payments system based on per diem prices. The agreed budget is expressed as an expected volume of services in various categories and prices per item of service. This provides a method of dividing the actual payments to a hospital (which should equal the budget) between the various insured or their insurers. It also provides a continuing set of price signals in the market. Any surplus or deficit remaining at the end of the year is eliminated in the subsequent year by price adjustments. There is scope for hospitals to negotiate changes to volume between years. If, for example, volume exceeded the planned level for two years running, a hospital might persuade the sickness funds and insurers to adjust the budget accordingly.

Initially, global budgets were based on historic costs with: additions for inflation; additions for the revenue consequences of approved capital projects; and across-the-board deductions of 1 or 2% per annum for assumed productivity gains. This tended to penalise the more efficient hospitals. Since 1988 an effort has been made to equalise the costs of given functions across acute hospitals. A formula is used to estimate target costs for each hospital. Certain cost categories such as interest, depreciation and maintenance, which account for about 20% of costs, are kept out of the model. Of the remaining national costs, 25% are allocated according to a hospital's catchment population, 35% are allocated according to the number of specialties and beds in the hospital (determined by planning) and 40% are allocated according to numbers of admissions, patient days, day treatments and "first out" patient visits (negotiable with the insurers).

Under this formula, money follows the patient to the extent that changes to catchment populations and volume are agreed in the annual negotiations about budgets. According to the formula, one-third of hospitals have target allocations which differ by more than 8% from current expenditure. There is a plan to bring actual allocations into line with target allocations by 1992 in steps of 2% (Rutten and Freens, 1986; Groot, 1987; Vos, 1988; Maarse, 1989; Saltman and de Roo, 1989).

Wages for non-medical hospital employees have been decided by central bargaining between the representatives of hospitals and labour unions. This process is subject to government directives on the maximum annual growth of labour costs per employee, which leave some scope for bargaining about pay rates, hours of work, and fringe benefits.

Most hospital investment is private (85% of beds are private) and hospitals usually borrow from the banking system to finance acquisitions. Investments have been subject to planning approval by provincial government. If planning approval is given, depreciation and interest on new investments can be included in prices and are automatically covered by sickness funds. Until now, bank loans have been guaranteed by the government. Academic hospitals are public and their investments have been financed by government grants. Such investments have been written off as soon as they are made.

REGULATION

In a system based on private institutions and independent practitioners, reliance in determining the volume and price of services was originally placed on decentralised bargaining between individuals, insurers and providers. Since the mid-1970s, however, mainly because of unacceptably high rates of growth in expenditure, the government has become increasingly involved in detailed regulation of prices and volume (Lapré, 1988; Kirkman-Liff et al., 1988; Saltman and de Roo, 1989). The result is that both private and public sectors are now heavily regulated.

Although the government does not control the overall health care budget – legally, both the compulsory and voluntary insurance schemes remain open-ended – it does intervene in other ways, including:

- It publishes an annual health expenditure plan which carries considerable weight and has, for all practical purposes, assumed the role of an overall indicative budget (see, for example, Ministry of Health and Environmental Protection, 1982);
- It closely regulates the two compulsory insurance schemes and has become increasingly involved in regulating private insurers;
- The Central Agency for Health Care Tariffs, established by the government in 1982, exercises strong controls over the fees and charges set by providers for both private and public patients and oversees the setting of hospital budgets. It also tries to regulate doctors' incomes;

- There are selected volume controls over the numbers of physicians admitted to training and the numbers of GPs allowed to practice, and efforts to reduce hospital capacity. Since 1982, hospitals have not been allowed to expand unless such expansion had been planned by local government and approved by the Ministry;
- There are wage controls for non-medical employees;
- As mentioned above, the government has sought to apply quality controls in health care for many years, via medical inspectors and a system of hospital accreditation.

In addition, the government introduced a number of reforms during the 1980s, including:

- The introduction of regional health planning, in 1982;
- The establishment of global budgets for hospitals, in 1983;
- The ending of voluntary insurance for basic care with sickness funds, in 1986;
- The introduction of a standard sickness insurance with a set premium for certain groups of privately insured, in 1986;
- The start of the process of equalising global budgets for hospitals, in 1988;
- The mandating of private insurers to provide basic insurance at set premiums for additional groups of high-risk patients, in 1989.

THE GROWTH AND PERFORMANCE OF THE SYSTEM

Judging from the OECD's data base (OECD, 1987; Schieber and Poullier, 1989; Tables 10.1, 10.2 and 10.3 in Chapter 10), the Netherlands has high standards of health and fairly typical health expenditure for a country with a high standard of living. In 1983, it ranked respectively 6th and 4th among OECD countries for life expectancy at birth for men (73.0 years) and women (79.8 years).

At $1 041 per capita, health expenditure in 1987 was a little above the level which would be expected on the basis of a regression line for OECD countries associating health expenditure with GDP per capita, using PPP exchange rates (Schieber and Poullier, 1989). The share of GDP devoted to health care, having risen rapidly from 3.9% in 1960 to 6.0% in 1970, and 8.0% in 1980 has more or less stabilized in the 1980s (it was 8.0% in 1989). Its physicians and acute beds per capita seem fairly typical of OECD countries. However, it has relatively low consultation rates with physicians, a very low prescribing rate, a relatively low acute hospital admission rate and a relatively high average length of stay in acute hospitals (Table 10.2, Chapter 10).

Following the introduction of global budgets for hospitals, there was a sharp fall in the rate of growth of real expenditure in hospitals and a pronounced fall in admissions. There was also an increase in waiting lists for elective surgery. In 1982, Rutten and van der Werff (1982) reported that in general waiting lists did not exist. However, according to a sample survey in 1989, the average waiting time was about 11 weeks in gynaecology and urology and about 15 weeks in orthopaedics in the Netherlands (Lorsheijd and Takx, 1990).

Since the early 1980s the government has had considerable success in keeping the rate of increase of doctors' fees well below the rate of increase of the consumer price index, but the effect on overall cost-containment has been less pronounced because of increases in the numbers of doctors per capita and in volume of services per doctor, especially for specialists (Kirkman-Liff, 1989).

Nevertheless, the amount of consumer choice continues to compare favourably with systems organised on more integrated lines. According to a British doctor who has worked in a Dutch hospital, "In Britain ... quality of care is in certain respects 'inferior' to that provided by the Dutch system, not in terms of specific medical treatment nor of professional commitment, but in terms of the nature of the relationship between the 'providers' and 'recipients' and access of the latter to the system and its services" (Beck, 1988).

BACKGROUND TO RECENT REFORMS

As discussed above, the Netherlands has achieved high standards of health and universal access to medical care at a cost that seems to be only a little above what would be expected for a country with a high standard of living.

Nevertheless, various problems remain. Some of these are unavoidable and face all OECD countries. They include the ageing of the population and the expenditure pressures associated with developing medical technology. The percentage of the population 65 and over is expected to increase from 11.5 to 15.1 between 1980 and

2010 (OECD, 1987). Other problems are more amenable to remedies as they are concerned with the design of the health care system itself and the incentives inherent within it. Four areas of shortcomings have been identified as leading to the setting up of the Committee on the Structure and Financing of Health Care (the Dekker Committee) in March 1987 (Ministry of Welfare, Health and Cultural Affairs, 1988; van de Ven, 1989).

Uncoordinated financing structure

Because there are several funders of health care who may be responsible for the same client at different points in an episode of illness, and because there are different funders of health and social services, there are barriers to substitution at critical points and a tendency for some providers to try to offload patients on other providers.

Health insurance

Various difficulties exist because of the partition of the health insurance system into four types. There is a lack of freedom of choice between the different insurance schemes, some difficulties in transition between them, and some remaining unfairness is perceived, especially the ability of the (young and healthy) privately insured to enjoy lower premiums than the better-off compulsorily insured because of their low risk and their freedom to rely on self-insurance. In the last 10 years, there has been a rapidly widening divergence in premiums in the private market reflecting the differences in risks.

Lack of incentives for efficiency

There are few *financial* incentives for consumers, insurers or producers to act efficiently. Consumers insured with sickness funds benefit from virtually free health care and have no incentives to restrain their demands. The sickness funds are reimbursed from a general fund for all realised claims expenses and consequently have no financial incentive to select efficient providers. Moreover, they are obliged to enter into contracts with any local provider who wishes to provide services to their members. This means that they act as passive funders of care rather than as active, cost-effective purchasers of services. Private insurers are more cost-conscious, but they find it easier to compete by avoiding enrolling individuals who represent poor risks than by choosing cost-effective providers. This is reinforced by the fact that their policy holders tend to enjoy free choice of provider. GPs are paid by capitation and have incentives to refer to specialists patients whom they might treat themselves. Specialists are paid by fee-for-service and are rewarded for unnecessary as well as necessary care. Because hospitals are now paid by global budgets it is arguable that they have inadequate incentives to respond to changes in demand. This dichotomy in incentives induces considerable tension between the specialists and hospital managers.

Government regulation

Imposed upon this system is a complex and highly centralised apparatus of government regulation of prices, volume and quality. This has been used with some success to restrain overall expenditure growth in recent years (despite the lack of an overall budget) but regulation is complex, costly, rigid and is forced to work against the grain of the system. It is difficult to co-ordinate the planning system with the financing system since they are the responsibility of different organisations and tend to conflict with each other.

These problems have manifested themselves in unacceptable cost pressures, excessive hospital expenditure compared with primary care expenditure and inexplicable variations between regions and sickness funds in health expenditure per capita. Against this background, the Dekker Committee was asked by the government to advise on:

- Strategies for volume and cost-containment against the background of an ageing population;
- A review of the finance and insurance system; and
- The possibilities for deregulation and streamlining within the health care system.

In its report, *Willingness to Change* (Ministry of Welfare, Health and Cultural Affairs, 1988), the Dekker Committee stated that it had adopted a number of starting points:

– The need for better integration of the financing and provision of care, especially across the health and related personal social services;
– The need for a move away from government regulation towards reliance on market forces;
– The maintenance of equity and solidarity.

The Committee proposed reforms under three main headings:

– Basic insurance covering both health and social services;
– Competition in the insurance market; and
– Competition in the provider market.

It may be noted, however, that no direct competition has been proposed in the ''market'' between patients and providers of care.

Chart 7.2 provides a summary of the reforms. At the heart of the proposals would be a system of compulsory basic insurance covering the bulk of both health and social services and accounting for about 85% of expenditure on these services. In addition, there would be voluntary supplementary insurance covering services such as drugs, dental care for adults, cosmetic surgery and abortion.

Competition in the insurance market was to be encouraged by the way in which the reformed insurance schemes would be designed. An ingenious feature of the basic insurance scheme was that the individual would pay a two-part premium, partly income-related and partly flat-rate. The bulk of the premium (about 75%) would be income-related at a rate fixed by the government and would be paid into a central fund. The central fund would then pay a risk-related premium to the competing insurer chosen by the individual. The rest of the premium (about 25%) would be flat-rate and would be paid direct by the individual to the insurer. Here, each insurer would be required to charge the same fixed rate to each subscriber, but the rate could differ between insurers. This would provide insurers with an incentive to compete to keep the flat-rate levy as low as possible and the quality of benefits as high as possible. Insurers would be obliged to accept all applicants. Meanwhile, because of the risk-related contribution from the central fund, the incentive for the insurer to compete on the basis of the individual's risk would be more or less eliminated. The distinction between sickness funds and private insurers would disappear.

Supplementary insurance would be voluntary. Insurers would be obliged to take all applicants, but the Committee felt that the government should only be drawn into the determination of insurance premiums if certain limits were exceeded.

The Committee envisaged that competition among insurers would encourage competition among providers. To promote such competition, the requirement for sickness funds to conclude a contract with all providers who sought one would be abolished. This would clear the way for insurers to select the most efficient providers of care.

The Committee also proposed a number of other measures, including a reduction of 4 000 hospital beds over four years, partial introduction of fees for some GP services, freeing-up of investment controls on hospitals and enhanced central encouragement and monitoring of mechanisms to ensure quality of care. There would also be reforms of certain advisory bodies.

Finally, the Committee made it clear that, whereas it regarded market mechanisms as the best way to promote efficiency in the health care system, it considered that the role of such mechanisms was limited by considerations of a social, cultural, ethical and economic nature. Government regulation would still be required, particularly where quality, cost control and equity were concerned. Care would also have to be taken to avoid abuse of monopoly power. What the Committee sought was a new balance among market forces, ethical principles and central regulation.

The publication of the Dekker report led to widespread and vigorous debate in the Netherlands (Ministry of Welfare, Health and Cultural Affairs, 1988; Schut and van de Ven, 1987). The government called public hearings in May 1987. Although much appreciation was expressed for the Committee's work, many doubts were raised also, including:

– Fears about risk selection and risk-related premiums for supplementary insurance;
– Concerns about the effect of flat-rate premiums for basic insurance on the poor and about the effect of income-related premiums for basic insurance on the rich; and

Chart 7.2 The health and social care system in the Netherlands following the Dekker reforms

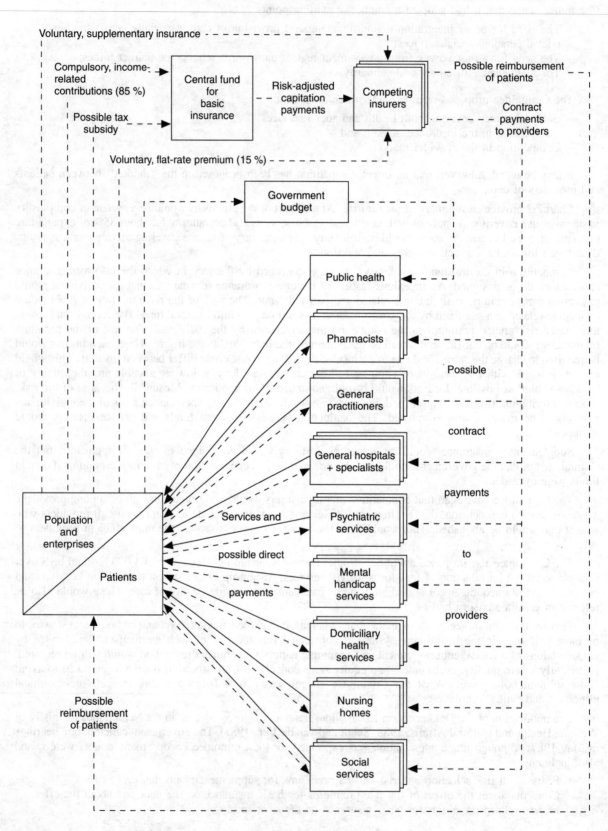

– Worries about the effect on costs of relaxation of government regulation in favour of reliance on market forces.

It was not until March 1988 that the then government felt able to put forward definite proposals for reform in a policy document entitled "Change Assured" which effectively endorsed the bulk of the Committee's proposals. More specifically the policy document confirmed the government's intention to proceed towards a unified system of compulsory basic health insurance for all the population; agreed that the role of market forces should be strengthened; and indicated that the extent of government regulation in the health care system should be reduced. The government's proposed reforms differed to some extent from those proposed by the Dekker Committee. In particular, it was decided to extend the package of basic insurance to include artificial aids and appliances. Also, insurers providing supplementary insurance would be obliged not only to accept new policy holders, but to charge all policy holders the same rate of premium, for any given level of risk-sharing.

Turning to the relationship between the insurers and the providers, the government stated that it saw these relationships as being largely contractual and a matter for free negotiation. Insurers would be free to refuse to conclude a contract with a provider. The minimum level of care to be provided under basic insurance would be described in legislation. The government felt that there was no need to set a maximum level of care. It anticipated that competition between insurers and the partial funding of insurers from the Central Fund by weighted capitation rather than by actual expenses would ensure that the provision of care developed in a "controlled" manner. Most planning and investment controls could be scrapped, but controls might have to be retained on capacity in large-scale residential institutions. Central guarantees for hospital investment loans would be scrapped. Capital charges would be established for academic hospitals to put them on the same basis as private hospitals. It would be necessary to put hospital depreciation on a replacement-cost basis. Determination of the level of prices could be left to the market, for the most part, but it would be necessary to prevent the development and abuse of monopolies and cartels.

On the key relationship between providers and those seeking care, the government saw quality and an improvement of the way the actual care is geared toward the needs and demands of patients as the main issues. These would be the responsibility of insurers and providers in the first instance, but the ultimate responsibility for the quality of the health care system lay with the government. There was a continuing role for the State Inspectorate and forthcoming legislation would be aimed at promoting the quality of professional practice. So far as the consumer was concerned, individuals should be given more opportunity to assert their independence while being protected in situations where they were inevitably dependent on another party.

There would remain an important role for the government itself in setting quality standards, in ensuring access for everyone and in controlling costs. In relation to costs, the government would retain powers to define the basic insurance package, to fix the amount of the income-related basic insurance premium, to control institutional capacity and to regulate prices and competition.

It would be necessary to implement the transition to the new system gradually, however, to smooth the impact on incomes of different households; to ensure that the appropriate legislation and administrative instruments were in place; and to enable a learning process to take place. A detailed timetable with four separate phases of action was set out with a view to completing the transition by 1992 (Ministry of Welfare, Health and Cultural Affairs, 1988).

The first stages of the reform were started in 1989. The exceptional medical expenses scheme was used as a vehicle for setting up the basic insurance scheme. The coverage of the scheme was extended to cover psychiatric care and artificial aids and appliances in January 1989. In addition, a small nominal premium was introduced for households enrolled with sickness funds.

Further implementation of the reforms was suspended for about six months while a new, centre-left government reconsidered the reforms. In May 1990 the new Cabinet announced that it would continue, albeit more slowly than had been envisaged previously, with the main thrust of the reforms (*Tweede Kamer der Staten-Generaal,* 1990). Some important changes were proposed, however. These changes were based on policy considerations (in order to encourage substitution between different types of services, the basic insurance was to cover all essential care) but also on legal requirements originating in international treaties (ILO and others) as well as European Community regulations. As a consequence,

– The content of the basic insurance package would be enlarged to cover about 90-95% of total health care expenditures (instead of 85%). The content of complementary insurance, which would be privately funded, would be correspondingly restricted.
– The ratio between the compulsory, income-related part of the premium for basic insurance and the negotiable flat-rate part would be 85/15 instead of 75/25.

- The writing of basic insurance would be restricted to non-profit insurers (because of European Community regulations).
- The first step would be to introduce in 1991 more competition into the sickness fund system by: introducing budgets for sickness funds; allowing sickness funds to decide nominal premiums for themselves; encouraging consumer choice between sickness funds; and making a start with the abolition of the duty of sickness funds to contract with each physician.
- The timetable for the reforms was extended, with full implementation envisaged as no earlier than 1995 (instead of 1992).

DISCUSSION

Potential benefits of reforms

Although the Dekker proposals can be traced back through van de Ven (1983 and 1987) to Enthoven's Consumer Choice Health Plan (Enthoven, 1980), they are striking for their originality. The model of financing and delivery (see Chart 7.2) must be regarded as a new variant which is not yet represented in other OECD countries, although the choice of an indemnity plan or an HMO option under Medicare in the United States bears some resemblance. The main innovation is the central fund for basic insurance which is intended to allow free consumer choice of insurer to be combined with compulsory finance. This amounts to a sophisticated health voucher scheme. Given competition among providers, it means that the relationship between insurers and providers could evolve along several different lines, depending on market forces.

The potential benefits of these reforms are considerable. They offer the prospect of significant improvements both in efficiency and in equity. This would be achieved by:

- Increasing consumers' choice of insurance cover and insurer;
- Encouraging insurers to be active purchasers;
- Giving providers competitive incentives to produce cost-effective care;
- Changing government's role from a direct regulator of price and volume to a facilitator of competitive markets;
- Enhancing government's control over total expenditure;
- Basing contributions more widely on ability to pay while retaining treatment according to need.

The reformed system has been carefully designed to overcome the two major weaknesses in voluntary health insurance: the tendencies of competing insurers to try to shun poor risks, and for insurance itself to encourage excessive growth of health expenditure. Risk selection will be countered mainly by the device of the central fund for basic insurance which will take in, from households and employers, premiums related to income and will pay out, to competing insurers, premiums related to the risk of their subscribers.

Excessive growth of expenditure will be discouraged by:

- The exposure of households to the voluntary, flat-rate premiums covering part of the cost of basic insurance (note: this does not in itself involve cost-sharing at the time when care is needed);
- Government control of the rate of compulsory contributions to the Central Fund which will account for the bulk of health and social service expenditure.

A further potential benefit of the reforms is the scope they provide for the development of such innovative health delivery systems such as "preferred provider organisations" and "health maintenance organisations" (van de Ven, 1988). Experience with such arrangements in the United States suggests that, compared with traditional open-choice, fee-for-service insurance, they can reduce costs without reducing quality.

Finally, a study into how the reforms will affect the equity of the financing of health care suggests that the current system is regressive and that, at best, this will be reduced, or, at the very least, remain unchanged (van Doorslaer *et al.*, forthcoming).

POTENTIAL DIFFICULTIES

There is, as yet, little experience of managed competition in the Netherlands or elsewhere. What difficulties are likely to arise in introducing the concept into the market for health insurance as well as for services?

The market for insurance

Some argue that the main problems are likely to be encountered in introducing managed competition into the market for health insurance. There are perhaps three potential difficulties here: risk selection; the formation of private monopsonies and cartels among insurers; and the possibility that the negotiable nominal premium, which is intended to account for 15% of the total premium for basic insurance, will be pushed upwards rather than downwards by competition.

On the question of risk selection, the scheme requires risk adjustment for individuals rather than for large groups, for which the law of large numbers applies. If the risk adjustments were too crude, the danger would be that insurers would put their competitive energies into "cream skimming" rather than into the search for more efficient care. The published documentation has not yet provided details as to how the risk adjustments will be made. However, Dutch health insurance data on individuals and data from the national Health Interview Survey show that, if the adjustments were based only on parameters such as age, gender and place of residence, insurers would still have a strong incentive to select some members of the population in favour of others. Such factors account for only about 20% of the non-random variation in health expenditure between individuals, whereas adding past health expenditures (which are readily available to insurers) accounts for about 60% of the non-random variation (van Vliet and van de Ven, 1990). Adding chronic sickness status accounts for about another 15% of the variation. For these reasons, it seems likely that longer-term expenses should be included in the distribution formula.

In addition, various types of pro-competitive regulation can be deployed to discourage cream skimming including: open enrolment; allowing, within limits, differentiation of the voluntary, flat-rate part of the basic insurance premium on grounds of risk; risk-sharing between the Central Fund and the insurers; and the promulgation of ethical codes for insurers. There seems a good prospect that some combination of these measures will be adequate to combat risk selection.

The inclusion of long-term health and social care in the basic insurance package puts a heavy strain on the mechanisms designed to avoid risk selection. The argument in favour of such inclusion is that it will help the integration and substitution of services across acute and long-term care, but against this it can be pointed out that long-term care is only an insurable risk *ex ante* and that it is a comparatively rare and distant event for most consumers. Also, given the association between low income and the need for long-term care, there is often a large distributional element in decisions about the level of care to be provided. Partly for these reasons, debate continues about whether long-term care should be covered in the basic insurance package or whether it should be covered in some other way – for example, by direct payments from the Central Fund.

A second worry must be about private monopoly and cartels in the market for insurance. Some concentration is desirable in the face of monopoly power among providers, but too much concentration in the market for insurance could put health insurers in a position to reduce benefits or raise the price of insurance. Although it is essential only that there be a *threat* of competition for markets to work efficiently, nevertheless the government (and courts) may have to work hard to preserve an appropriate competitive environment, especially in view of mergers between insurers (Schut, 1990).

The third concern is that the voluntary, flat-rate part of the insurance premium may be competed upwards rather than downwards. This could happen if sufficient consumers were persuaded that it was worth paying for a higher volume or quality of care than the government was willing to finance through the Central Fund. In general, private health insurance markets show a considerable propensity for rising premiums, even in the absence of government subsidies, and the new market would be subsidised to the tune of about 85% of the initial average premiums. Rising nominal premiums would be inefficient if they encouraged unnecessary care, but the most obvious threat they would pose would be to equity. It is even possible to envisage that some insurers might try to corner the market for certain medical care resources in inelastic supply, such as senior specialist doctors.

The market for services

There are several concerns here, including the risk that competition could take place to the detriment of quality of care and the possibility that providers might exploit monopoly power. There are arguments for keeping concern about quality in perspective, the most important of which is that competition will itself provide incentives for insurers and providers to offer (and maintain) quality of care because otherwise they will risk placing themselves at a competitive disadvantage (van de Ven, 1989). However, the difficulty which consumers (and governments) have in judging quality is well known in health care. No one doubts that competing providers will have an incentive to present an *image* of high quality care, but it is the *reality* that will matter. Fortunately, the Netherlands already has well-developed institutions for quality insurance initiated both by the government and by the providers themselves (Giebing, 1987; Kistemaker, 1987; Reerink, 1987). There will be strong pressures on insurers to demonstrate that quality assurance is pursued by the providers with whom they have contracts. In addition, it is hoped that in the new climate of consumer choice, bodies representing consumers' interests, such as private certification institutes, will spring up to measure quality (van de Ven, 1989).

There will undoubtedly be a need to avoid the abuse of monopoly power in provider markets. Providers in the Netherlands have traditionally formed strong professional associations and various open and tacit agreements in restraint of trade. Many hospitals possess some monopoly power on account of their specialisation and geographical location. Until now, government policy has often reinforced such arrangements. In future it will be necessary to adopt pro-competitive regulation, especially since the insurers will not be public monopsonies. As with insurers, there are reports that hospitals have been merging (Schut, 1990).

Transition to the new system

Finally, perhaps the most difficult problem will be how to effect the transition to the reformed system. The government has, on several occasions, extended the timetable for legislative and administrative action to achieve phased change (*Tweede Kamer der Staten-Generaal,* 1990). In March 1992, a kind of temporary freeze on new changes to the system came into force pending a public review by parliament in September-October 1992. Consultative papers were tabled by the government to promote further quality assurance and to streamline the existing consultative machinery. A number of mergers of private and public insurers took place with some for-profit insurers shedding their health insurance portfolio. Following the insertion of pharmaceutical coverage in the ABZW scheme which is the vehicle chosen for the new basic insurance, pharmaceutical consumption of some population segments augmented rapidly, bringing cost-containment once again as a main item on the agenda. It is still too early to gauge the reaction of the other participants in the process – consumers, insurers and providers – and, indeed, the evolution of the political process itself in a pluralistic society (Elsinga, 1989). Although the omens look good – not least because of the basis of private institutions which already exists – it will be some years before it will be known whether the reforms have proceeded to fulfil their promise.

References

Ballay, U. (1990), "Dutch Health Reforms in the 1980s", *Health Services Management,* February.

Beck, E. J. (1988), "An Anglo-Dutch Comparison of Health Care Delivery – The Return of the Prodigal Son", *Community Medicine,* Vol. 10, No. 1.

Elsinga, E. (1989), "Political decision-making in health care – the Dutch case", *Health Policy,* 11, pp. 243-255.

Enthoven, A. C. (1980), *Health Plan: The Only Practical Solution to the Soaring Cost of Health Care,* Addison Wesley.

Giebing, H. A. (1987), "Unit-based Approach for Nursing Quality Assurance in the Netherlands: one year experience", *Australian Clinical Review,* March.

Groot, L. M. J. (1987), "Incentives for Cost-Effective Behaviour: A Dutch Experience", *Health Policy,* Vol. 7.

Heuvel, W. J. A., van den (1990), "Developments in Dutch Health Care Policy: The Ideology of Market Mechanism", *Cah. Socio. Demo. Med.* 30(3), July-September.

Kirkman-Liff, B. L. (1989), "Cost-Containment and Physician Payment Methods in the Netherlands", *Inquiry,* Vol. 26, Winter.

Kirkman-Liff, B. L., Lapré, R. and Kirkman-Liff, T. L. (1988), "The Metamorphosis of Health Planning", *Journal of Health Planning and Management,* Vol. 3.

Kirkman-Liff, B. L. and van de Ven, W. P. M. M. (1989), "Improving Efficiency in the Dutch Health Care System", *Health Policy,* Vol. 13.

Kistemaker, W. J. G. (1987), "Peer Review in the Hospitals of the Netherlands", *Australian Clinical Review,* March.

Lapré, R. (1988), "A change of direction in the Dutch health care system?", *Health Policy* 10, pp. 21-32.

Lorsheijd, J. J. G., and Takx, O. P. (1990), "Enquete toont: wachtlijsten niet alleen voor dure ingrepen", *Het Ziekenhuis,* pp. 5-15, March.

Maarse, J. A. M. (1989), "Hospital Budgeting in Holland: aspects, trends and effects", *Health Policy,* 11, pp. 257-276.

Ministry of Health and Environmental Protection (1982), *Health Care in the Netherlands: Financial Analysis 1976-1983,* September.

Ministry of Welfare, Health and Cultural Affairs (1988), *Changing health care in the Netherlands,* September.

Ministry of Welfare, Health and Cultural Affairs (1989), *Health Insurance in the Netherlands,* September.

OECD (1987), *Financing and Delivering Health Care,* Paris.

Posthuma, B. H., van der Zee, J. and Gloerich, F. B. M. (1990), "(Cost) Effects of Private Health Insurance Options; the Case of the Netherlands", paper presented at the Second World Congress in Health Economics, Zurich, September.

Reerink, E. (1987), "Quality Assurance in the Health Care System in the Netherlands", *Australian Clinical Review,* March.

Roo, A. A. de (1988), "Netherlands", in *The International Handbook of Health Care Systems,* Edited by Saltman, R. B., Greenwood Press, New York.

Rutten, F. F. H. (1987), "Market Strategies for publicly Financed Health Care Systems", *Health Policy,* Vol. 7.

Rutten, F. F. H. and Freens, R. J. M. (1986), "Health Care Financing in the Netherlands: recent changes and future options", *Health Policy,* 6, pp. 313-320.

Rutten, F. F. H. and van der Werff, A. (1982), "Health policy in the Netherlands", *The Public/Private Mix for Health,* Ed., McLachlan G. and Maynard A., Nuffield Provincial Hospitals Trust.

Saltman, R. B. and de Roo, A. A. (1989), "Hospital Policy in the Netherlands: the Parameters of Structural Stalemate", *Journal of Health Politics, Policy and Law,* Vol. 14, No. 4, Winter.

Sandier, S. (1990), "Health Services Utilisation and Physician Income Trends", in *Health Care Systems in Transition,* OECD, Paris.

Schieber, G. J. and Poullier, J.-P. (1989), "International Health Care Expenditure Trends: 1987", *Health Affairs,* Fall.

Schieber, G. J. Poullier, J. P., and Greenwald, L. M., Health Care Systems in Twenty-Four Countries, *Health Affairs,* Fall.

Schut, F. T. (1990), "Prospects for Workable Competition in Health Care: Dutch Design and American Experience", paper presented at the Second World Congress on Health Economics, Zurich, September.

Schut, F. T. and van de Ven, W. P. M. M. (Editors) (1987), *Proceedings of the Conference on Regulated Competition in the Dutch Health Care System,* Erasmus University, Rotterdam, November.

Tiddens, H. A., Heesters, J. P. and van de Zande, J. M. (1984), "Health services in the Netherlands", in Raffel, M.W., *Comparative Health Systems,* Pennsylvania State University Press.

Tweede Kamer der Staten-Generaal (1990), *Werken aan Zorgvernieuwing, Vergaderjaar 1989-1990,* 21 545, No. 1.

van de Ven, W. P. M. M. (1983), "Ziektekostenverzekering en financiele prikkels tot doelmatigheid", *Economische Statistische Berichten,* p. 68, 72-78 and 110-117.

van de Ven, W. P. M. M. (1987), "The key role of health insurance in a cost-effective health care system", *Health Policy,* Vol. 7.

van de Ven, W. P. M. M. (1988), "A future for competitive health care in the Netherlands", paper prepared for the congress, "A future for the competitive health care in Europe?", June 20-22, 1988, Rotterdam, Revised November.

van de Ven, W. P. M. M. (1989), "Health insurance reforms and incentives", paper prepared for the European Conference on Health Economics, Barcelona, 19-21 September.

van de Ven, W. P. M. M. (1990), "From Regulated Cartel to Regulated Competition in the Dutch Health Care System", *European Economic Review,* Vol. 34.

van de Ven, W. P. M. M. and van Vliet, R. C. J. A. (1990), "How can we prevent cream skimming in a competitive health insurance market?", paper presented at the Second World Congress on Health Economics, Zurich, September.

van Doorslaer, E. K. A., Janssen, R. T. J. M., Wagstaff, A., van Emmerik, J. P. M. et Rutten, F. F. H. (forthcoming), "Equity in the Finance of Health Care: Effects of the Dutch Health Insurance Reform", in *Proceeding of First European Conference on Health Economics,* Berlin, Springer Verlag.

van Vliet, R. C. J. A. and van de Ven, W. P. M. M. (1990), "Towards a Budget Formula for Competing Health Insurers", paper presented at the Second World Congress on Health Economics, Zurich, September.

Vos, B. (1988), *Uncertainty in Funding: Consequences for Hospital Management,* National Hospital Institute, Utrecht, May.

Chapter 8

THE REFORM OF THE HEALTH SYSTEM OF SPAIN[1]

INTRODUCTION

During the 1980s, the Spanish government introduced major changes to its health care system, involving the consolidation of a national health system. The main reforms included the extension of compulsory health insurance from about 90% to virtually the entire population; better planning and integration of both primary and hospital care; increased reliance on funding out of general taxation; and the beginning of the devolution of health care administration to the autonomous regions.

This chapter describes a health care system which before (and, indeed, after) the reforms contained a complex mixture of public and private financing and public and private provision. The chapter goes on to consider some of the problems which gave rise to the reforms and then provides a summary account of the most important reforms. The growth and performance of the system is then described. Finally, some remaining weaknesses in the provision of health care and a major new report on the system are discussed.

HEALTH CARE SYSTEM BEFORE THE REFORMS

As with other health care systems, it is possible to discern a number of historical layers, incompletely co-ordinated, in the Spanish health care system. By 1980, however, the system was already dominated by a compulsory health insurance system, *Instituto Nacional de la Salud* (INSALUD), which was part of the social security system, and by public primary health care arrangements and public hospitals. Public primary care and the bulk of public general hospitals were organised according to the integrated model (see Chapter 2) but there was also considerable contracting between INSALUD and various public and private non-INSALUD clinics and hospitals. This compulsory system was supplemented by considerable voluntary health expenditure made up of both direct payments and private health insurance.

Chart 8.1 provides a summary description of the system before the reforms. At the bottom left is the population, most of whom become patients in any one year. At the bottom right are the providers. At the top are the third party payers, including INSALUD and private insurers. Service flows are shown as solid lines, financial flows as broken lines.

The providers have been divided into public health services (including mental health care), independent pharmacists, primary health care clinics in rural areas, general practitioners and non-hospital specialists, private medical practices, INSALUD hospitals, other public hospitals, and private hospitals. Dentists have been excluded from the diagram, as have a range of private and public social services (nursing homes, residential homes and domiciliary services) which are financed mainly by another branch of social security (INSERSO) or by private expenditure.

The third-party payers are dominated by INSALUD, the health branch of the social security system, and by various statutory schemes for civil servants which between them accounted for about 68% of all health expenditure and which covered 90% of the population in 1980. Other tax-funded programmes accounted for about 8% of expenditure. Voluntary health insurance (mainly for the self-employed in 1980) accounted for about 3% of all health expenditure.

Apart from pharmaceuticals, there is no cost-sharing in the public sector of the health care system. Nevertheless, voluntary direct payments, mainly for ambulatory, medical, dental and pharmaceutical care and for appliances, play an important role, representing about 21% of all health expenditure in 1980.

Chart 8.1 Major service and financial flows in the Spanish health care system before the reforms

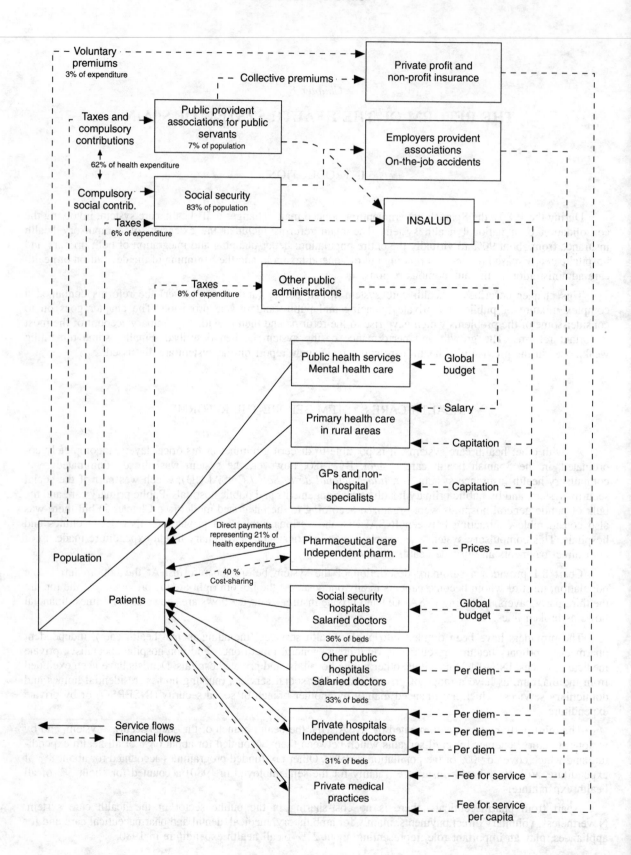

Voluntary premiums
3% of expenditure

Collective premiums

Private profit and non-profit insurance

Taxes and compulsory contributions

Public provident associations for public servants
7% of population

Employers provident associations
On-the-job accidents

62% of health expenditure

Compulsory social contrib.

Social security
83% of population

INSALUD

Taxes
6% of expenditure

Taxes
8% of expenditure

Other public administrations

Public health services
Mental health care

Global budget

Primary health care in rural areas

Salary

Capitation

GPs and non-hospital specialists

Capitation

Population

Patients

Direct payments representing 21% of health expenditure

40 % Cost-sharing

Pharmaceutical care
Independent pharm.

Prices

Social security hospitals
Salaried doctors
36% of beds

Global budget

Other public hospitals
Salaried doctors
33% of beds

Per diem

Private hospitals
Independent doctors
31% of beds

Per diem
Per diem
Per diem

Fee for service

Private medical practices

Fee for service per capita

Service flows
Financial flows

Ambulatory care

Prior to the reforms, there were three main routes to ambulatory medical care and a three-tier referral system in the public sector. First, patients insured by INSALUD could register with a general practitioner (GP) chosen from a panel, with limited opportunities for changing doctors. The GPs tended to work in INSALUD clinics, at least in urban areas. Second, patients on low incomes, not covered by INSALUD, could go to a physician working under contract with the local municipality. In both cases, the GP might refer patients to a specialist in an ambulatory clinic, where the specialists would not have direct access to hospital beds. Such specialists might then refer the patient to a hospital. However, GPs and specialists in the public sector were linked in a pyramidal system which constrained the gatekeeper's choice of specialist to a list of specialists which served the locality. Third, those able to pay could go to a GP for a private consultation, or directly to a specialist, avoiding the GP gatekeeper. Many doctors worked part-time, having more than one public post and a private practice. Since the reforms, public ambulatory care is increasingly based on full-time, primary health care teams consisting of GPs, paediatricians and nurses in public health centres which serve a defined geographical area, and on full-time specialists based in hospital out-patient departments. A restricted choice of specialist remains.

Doctors who treat public patients are free to prescribe drugs, which are usually dispensed by independent pharmacists. Generally, the patient has to meet 40% of the cost of the drug. Pensioners are exempt from charges, as are patients who need certain life-saving drugs. The rest of the cost is paid directly by social security.

Hospital care

There are four main types of hospital: INSALUD hospitals with about 36% of beds (mainly general); provincial and municipal hospitals with about 33% of beds (many long-term); private non-profit hospitals with about 14% of beds; and private proprietary hospitals with about 17% of beds. There are no private beds in public hospitals. INSALUD has contracts for patient care with many non-INSALUD public and private hospitals. Indeed, although social security manages only 36% of beds, it finances between 75 and 80% of all hospital stays. INSALUD gives preference to public over private hospitals and to non-profit over for-profit hospitals. Direct payments for private hospital care are negligible.

Long-term care

Psychiatric hospitals were provided mainly by the provincial governments and by the Catholic Church. A network of new mental health centres and psychiatric units in general hospitals is now being set up under the national health system (Duran and Blanes, 1991). Separate social services provide various forms of institutional and domiciliary care, for the elderly and mentally ill, alongside private services.

RELATIONSHIP BETWEEN POPULATION AND THIRD-PARTY PAYERS

In 1980 about 83% of Spaniards were covered for comprehensive health care under INSALUD, with another 7% covered by the statutory schemes for civil servants and the armed forces. The schemes were financed mainly by compulsory social security contributions made by employees and employers. These were set at 39% of earnings in 1980 (33% employer and 6% employee) with a lower and an upper earnings limit. They covered pension contributions also. About 30% of social security contributions were allocated to INSALUD and there was a tax subsidy of about 10 %. Benefits were comprehensive, including GP, specialist, pharmaceutical and hospital care and dental extractions. The self-employed were free to make their own insurance arrangements; about one in three chose INSALUD, with the remainder choosing private insurers or no insurance at all.

Public employees were compulsorily insured under a scheme which allowed them to chose between INSALUD and private insurers and providers. About two-thirds chose private insurers.

Apart from the subsidy to the social security system, general taxation by central and local government accounted for about 8% of total health expenditure in 1980.

At the beginning of the decade, private insurance was chosen by most public employees and by certain groups, such as the self-employed, who were not required to join the statutory scheme. Voluntary private insurance accounted for only about 3% of health expenditure in 1980. Following the inclusion of the self-employed in the statutory scheme in 1984 – and the freeing of private insurers from the requirement to provide comprehensive insurance – voluntary health insurance has become increasingly supplementary, except for public employees. About 10% of Spaniards now carry both statutory and private health insurance. For tax purposes, 15% of private health expenditure and insurance premiums may be deducted from income.

Of the 200 or so private insurers – both commercial and non-profit – the six largest account for nearly half of the market. Among the commercial insurers are many small and local companies owned by physicians. These are similar to health maintenance organisations in the United States. Sometimes, the doctors are paid by capitation. The non-profit insurers include both *mutuelles* organised by professional groups and *igualatorios* managed by doctors' organisations on a co-operative basis. In this case, doctors are paid directly by fee for service, rather like independent practice associations in the United States. Spain does not have a strong tradition of reimbursement insurance. However, the market is changing with the entry of multi-national insurers.

RELATIONSHIPS BETWEEN THIRD-PARTY PAYERS AND PROVIDERS

Ambulatory care

In 1980, most GPs and many specialists were engaged by INSULAD in urban areas and both by INSALUD and by the municipalities in rural areas. They were paid by capitation by the former and by salary by the latter. GPs in urban areas and ambulatory care specialists engaged by INSALUD were required to work for two hours per day at the clinic at hours notified to their patients (usually in the morning) and to make home visits. GPs in rural areas provided a 24-hour service, most of them working in isolation. Under the new arrangements for primary health care teams, which are responsible for fixed catchment populations, doctors are salaried and work six hours daily. Doctors who provide independent ambulatory care may be paid by fee for service, but in the case of prepaid group practices, they often receive capitation payments.

Independent pharmacists are paid by fee for service. The price of drugs is subject to product-by-product bargaining between the Ministry of Health and the pharmaceutical companies. This is designed to award prices which, for the most part, are equal to or lower than the lowest price for the same or a similar product elsewhere in Europe (Young, 1990).

Hospitals

INSALUD hospitals are funded by a rigid system of global budgets which is based mainly on historical costs. Separate budgets exist for various types of operating cost and capital expenditure. Local managers do not have the freedom to use money granted under one budget to purchase items under another budget. Any savings made are automatically removed to a central INSALUD budget (Brooks, 1987). Capital expenditure is in the form of grants, with no subsequent payments for depreciation or interest. Hospitals which are contracted with INSALUD are paid per diem at rates which depend upon their functional classification. The rates cover capital charges for both public and private hospitals under contract.

Doctors in public hospitals are salaried and in private hospitals are paid by fee for service. Doctors in public hospitals cannot have private patients, but they are allowed to work part-time in the private sector. Since 1987, they have been given incentives to work full-time in the public sector.

Government regulation and planning

In keeping with its predominantly integrated nature, the Spanish health care system is highly regulated. At the beginning of the 1980s the system was also highly centralised through INSALUD. During the decade, however, there has been considerable devolution from the centre to the autonomous regions (this is discussed further below).

Central control is exercised in a variety of ways: legislation; the provision of funds; the salaried nature of most employment; global budgets; and public ownership of the bulk of clinics, health centres and hospitals. In addition, central government monitors the prescribing of drugs, negotiates drug prices, regulates the contracting out of patient care to hospitals, accredits hospitals and health centres, licenses independent facilities and sets a ceiling on the enrolment of medical students. Central and regional governments also regulate private health insurance.

BACKGROUND TO REFORMS

At the beginning of the 1980s, the health care system already demonstrated many strong points, including low rates of perinatal mortality, broad equity in access, a high level of acceptance by society, and a relatively low level of health expenditure. However, a number of weaknesses were perceived, including the following:

- Gaps existed in compulsory health insurance cover. The self-employed were able to escape compulsory contributions and the poorest members of society – for example, those who had never had a regular job – were excluded from the mainstream of care financed by INSALUD.
- Although the government had acquired considerable control over total spending, adverse cost pressures persisted. At the same time, complaints were being made about inadequate public spending on health care.
- It was generally felt that there were failings in the efficiency and quality of public sector services. These related less to the technical quality of services (although there was an absence of quality assurance) than to consumer satisfaction. Public ambulatory care was often seen as second class with long queues, hasty consultations (lasting, on average, three minutes with a GP and seven minutes with a specialist), and impersonal care. And while public hospitals were esteemed for their skilled staff and high-technology equipment, they often suffered from crowded emergency departments, lengthy in-patient waiting lists (four per 1 000 population), and a lack of comfort (Saturno, 1988).
- Considerable stresses and strains were evident at the complex and permeable boundaries between the public and private sectors. Doctors who provided ambulatory care, usually combined private practice with a public post. This gave them financial disincentives to improve their services to public patients (Miguel and Guillen, 1989; Rodriguez, Calonge and Rene, 1990). Meanwhile, access to private, ''first class'' care was governed by ability to pay.
- The public system was seen as fragmented, poorly co-ordinated, over-bureaucratic, over-centralised and under-managed (Brooks, 1987).
- Doubts were expressed over the allocation of resources: in particular, in comparison with other OECD countries, Spain appeared to have too many doctors and a shortage of hospital beds (see below). The excess of doctors was associated with medical unemployment and relatively low pay.

REFORMS OF THE EIGHTIES

Chart 8.2 depicts the health care system following the reforms. Because some of the more important reforms are being introduced only gradually, the chart is not dated. For example, only about half of the proposed primary health care teams have been established so far.

Major reforms

The main reforms to the health care system during the 1980s were as follows:

1981: Catalonia became the first autonomous region to be responsible for its own health care system under social security.

1984: The self-employed were brought into compulsory health insurance and private insurers were released from the requirement to provide only comprehensive cover.

1984: A start was made on the reform of primary health care. This involved the creation of primary health care teams with full-time salaried doctors and nurses based on health centres serving a defined geographical area.

1986: The General Health Law was passed creating a national health system. This involved:

- Providing for the decentralisation of INSALUD to all the autonomous regions with a view to creating 17 regional health services within a national system.
- The incorporation of provincial, municipal and social security health services (including mental health services) in an integrated network.
- Legislative support for the primary health care reforms started in 1984.
- The setting up of supra-regional health Council with the aim of co-ordinating policy and planning between the different regional health services.

The Law also confirmed the right to free practice of the health professions, and freedom of enterprise for private clinics and hospitals, subject to licensing by the health authorities.

Chart 8.2 Major service and financial flows in the Spanish health care system after the reforms

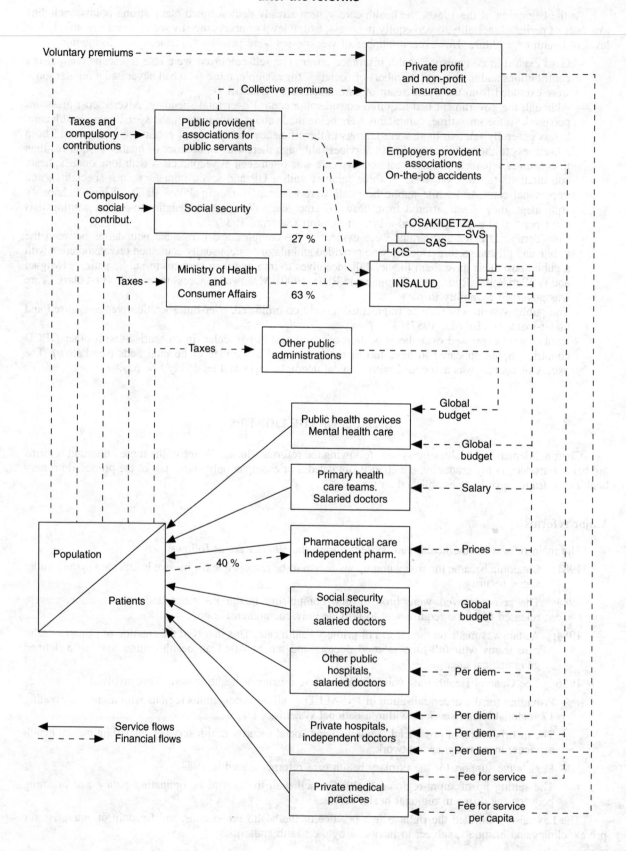

1986-1987: Extension of health insurance under social security to include the remaining uninsured dependent relatives of contributors.

1987: Public hospital doctors were given financial incentives to work full-time for the public sector opportunities to earn productivity bonuses.

1989: The indigent poor were made eligible for mainstream INSALUD cover subject to a means test.

1989: Changing the basis for financing the system. There would be shift towards general taxation. From 1989 the social security contribution rate for health care would be fixed, leaving general taxation to take up the residual (it was 73 % in 1989). This would presumably make the funding of the system more progressive.

Other reforms

Other significant reforms were as follows.

1979: A ceiling was placed on the intake of medical students to medical schools.

1981: Catalonia introduced an accreditation procedure for hospital services.

1985: A start was made on strengthening the management function in hospitals and on improving management information.

1985: A Central Commission on Quality Assurance was set up in support of confidential peer review in public hospitals.

1986: Quality assurance was introduced into primary care.

1987: A law was passed on the reorganisation of the management of INSALUD.

1991: A negative list for drugs was introduced. Steps were also taken towards creating a more competitive market for pharmaceuticals.

1992: Within the framework of a government strategy of European convergence, decision to move towards a greater autonomy of hospitals, converted into quasi-public corporations.

GROWTH AND PERFORMANCE

According to OECD figures, the share of health expenditure in GDP rose from 2.3% in 1960 to 4.1% in 1970 and to 6.6% in 1990. A rise of 1% occurred in the share between 1980 and 1990, against a 2% rise in GDP itself.

Per capita health expenditure in 1987 was $521 denominated in US$ using GDP purchasing power parity exchange rates. This was just below the expected level according to a regression analysis linking per capita health expenditure with per capita GDP for OECD countries (Schieber and Poullier, 1989).

The data recorded in OECD (1987), in Schieber et al. (1991) and in Table 10.2, suggest that Spain has had more doctors per capita but fewer hospital beds than most other OECD countries. Acute hospital bed days per capita and acute hospital admissions are among the lowest recorded in the OECD and acute hospital length of stay is also below average. Consultations with doctors per capita are also below average, but the figures, here, exclude the private sector. Prescribed drugs per capita are slightly above the OECD average.

Average life expectancy at birth was 79.7 years for females and 73.3 years for males in 1985. These figures were respectively equal to and above the highest average life expectancy recorded by the other six countries in this study. However, Le Grand (1987) has shown that, after age standardization, Spain had a greater dispersion in age of death than any of the other six countries, except perhaps France, depending on the precise measure chosen. Such inequality in age of death is probably mainly a result of the underlying socio-economic inequities in Spanish society (Rodriguez and Lemkow, 1990). Perinatal mortality rates – 1.06% of births in 1987 – were lower than in Ireland but higher than in the other countries considered in this study. Because of the multi-causal nature of the determinants of mortality, however, it is not possible to draw any firm conclusions about the performance of the Spanish health care system from these data.

According to a survey conducted in 1991 only 21% of Spaniards were content with the working of their health system, although 71% of those who had actually received care were satisfied with the treatment they had received. These figures were lower than for the other countries included in this study (Blendon et al., 1991).

REMAINING PROBLEMS AND POTENTIAL SOLUTIONS

Despite its many strengths, the Spanish health care system still appears to suffer from problems in several areas. The formation of full-time, salaried, primary health care teams, which now cover about half of the population, will have raised standards in the public ambulatory care sector. The teams have increased the commitment of doctors and other primary care workers to public service and have encouraged continuity of care and prevention. However, it has been suggested that in some respects, the services are operating rather as before. and remain unresponsive to consumers. Judging by experience in Ireland, it may be satisfactory for higher income earners in Spain to continue to make their own arrangements for general and specialist medical care in the private sector. However, it is open to question whether Spain has found the best arrangements for securing the efficient provision of *public* ambulatory medical care.

Spain is the only one of the seven countries which aims to rely wholly on salaried service in the public sector, which allows patients to change their doctor only under special circumstances, and restricts the choice of specialist by the gatekeeper. Although such arrangements are capable of making available skilled public care to all who need it – free of charge to the patient and at a reasonable cost to the taxpayer –, they seem to foster a kind of captive market in favour of the provider and to encourage queues and a brisk and impersonal style of service. In short, the system does not respond well to consumer demands. It is interesting to speculate what would happen if – within the country's given budget for public ambulatory care – primary care providers were given an incentive to compete for patients as well as a chance to choose the specialists to whom they refer their patients.

Similar observations can be made about hospital services. In the case of INSALUD hospitals, global budgets, with clawback of any savings, are effective at containing costs to the level desired by the third-party payers. At the same time, however, budgets provide perverse incentives for efficiency. More effective providers are rewarded by increased work or smaller budgets, rather than by more money, and the less effective providers can be rewarded by a quieter life. Although a large part of hospital services are contracted out by INSALUD, the approach seems to be to award contracts on the basis of ownership rather than on that of efficiency. No reliance seems to be placed on competition among providers.

In 1990 the Parliament appointed a Commission on the analysis and Evaluation of the National Health System, which was to conduct a thorough review. The Commission issued its report (*Comision de Analisis y Evaluacion del Sistema Nacional de Salud,* 1991) a year later. Its diagnosis of problems in the national health system included: a lack of cost-consciousness among consumers; insufficient choice for patients in the public sector; and failures of efficiency, arising partly from inappropriate incentives, among providers. In making its recommendations, the Commission took care to stress that the equity and solidarity at the core of the system should not be disturbed. However, it advocated some radical reforms including:

- increasing the share of social security contributions in the financing of the system;
- defining basic (core) services more clearly and introducing extra payment for supplementary services;
- introducing nominal charges for certain basic services, including extending the 40% co-insurance payments for pharmaceuticals to pensioners;
- separating the purchasing and provision of hospital care, making the Health Areas, which had hitherto been responsible for primary care, the purchasers;
- improving management and management information in public hospitals;
- giving a considerable measure of self-government to public hospitals by transforming them into state-owned firms; and
- introducing more flexible, performance-related contracts for health service employees.

The report generated much controversy. In particular, there was a public outcry about the proposal to extend prescription charges to pensioners. More generally, the authors of the report were criticised: for copying major features of the reforms in the United Kingdom without adapting them adequately to Spanish circumstances; for saying little about improving choice in primary care; and for failing to address more directly what were perceived as critical weaknesses in the organisation, administration and management of the National Health System.

The government has promised not to implement the recommendations concerning drugs charges for pensioners and has postponed for several months taking decisions on most of the other recommendations in the report.

Note

1. This chapter is based on a paper prepared by J. Hernandez Pascual, Ministry of Health and Consumer Affairs, Madrid, who is therefore not responsible for opinions or errors in the final edited version.

References

Abel-Smith, B. (1984), *Cost-Containment in Health Care: the Experience of Twelve European Countries 1977-1983,* London, Bedford Square Press.

Artells Herrero, J.J., Rodriguez Artalejo, F., Palleja, P. and Hernandez Pascual, J. (1990), "Spain: Current Developments", paper delivered at a WHO meeting on New Approaches to Managing Health Services, Leeds, U.K., January.

Beaud, S. (1988), "La Protection Sociale en Espagne", *La Note de L'Ires,* No. 15, 1st Quarter.

Blendon, R.J. *et al.*, (1991), "Spain's Citizens Assess Their Health Care System", *Health Affairs,* Fall.

Brooks, A. (1987), "Administrator...in Name Only", *The Health Service Journal,* 3 September.

Comisíon de Análisis y Evaluacíon del Sistema Nacional de Salud (1991), *Informe y Recomendaciones,* Julio.

Duran, E. and Blanes, T. (1991), "Spain: Democracy followed by devolution", in *Mental Health Services in the Global Village,* Edited by Appleby, L. and Araya, R., Royal College of Psychiatrists, Gaskell.

Hernandez Pascual, J. (1989), "Private Health Insurance in Spain and the Integration of the European Market", paper delivered at a Meeting on Health Care in Europe after 1992, Erasmus University, Rotterdam, the Netherlands, October.

Ibern, P. (1990), "Trends and Evolution of the Spanish Health Care System", in *Competitive Health Care in Europe: Future Prospects,* Casparie, A.F. *et al.* (ed.), Dartmouth Publishing Co. Ltd.

Kelley, J.B. (1984), "Health Care in the Spanish Social Security System: Public-Private Relationships", *International Journal of Health Services,* Vol. 14, No. 2.

Laporte, J.-R., Porta, M., Capella, D. and Arnau J.M.(1984), "Drugs in the Spanish Health Care System", *International Journal of Health Services,* Vol. 14, No. 4.

Le Grand, J. (1987), "Inequalities in Health: Some International Comparisons", *European Economic Review,* Vol. 31, pp. 182-191.

Lopez Casasnovas, G. (1989), "La Reforma de Los Sistemas Nacionales de Salud", paper prepared for the First European Congress of Health Economics, Barcelona, September.

Miguel, J.M. de, and Guillen M.-F. (1989), "The Health System in Spain", in *Success and Crisis in National Health Systems,* Edited by Field, M.G., Routledge, New York.

Ministerio de Sanidad y Consumo (1989), *The Spanish Health System: Highlights,* Madrid.

OECD (1987), *Financing and Delivering Health Care,* OECD, Paris.

Rodriguez, M. (1990), "The Health Care System in Spain", *Competitive Health Care in Europe: Future Prospects,* Casparie, A.F. *et al.,* ed., Dartmouth Publishing Co. Ltd.

Rodriguez, J.A., and Lemkow, L. (1990), "Health and Social Inequities in Spain", *Social Science and Medicine,* Vol. 31, No. 31.

Rodriguez, M., Calonge, S. and Rene, J. (1990), "An Analysis of Equity in the Financing and Delivery of Health Care in Spain", discussion paper presented to the EEC COMAC Project on "Distributive Effects of Health Policies, Bellagio Conference, 12-16 November.

Rovira, J. (1987), ''Appraisal of a Proposal to Allow the Beneficiaries of the Social Security in Catalonia to Choose between Public and Private Health Care Provision'', paper delivered at a Meeting of the Health Economists Study Group, Newcastle Upon Tyne, United Kingdom, December.

Saturno, P.J. (1988), ''Spain'', in *The International Handbook of Health Care Systems,* Edited by Saltman, R.B., Greenwood Press, New York.

Schieber, G.J. and Poullier, J.-P. (1989), ''International Health Care Expenditure Trends'', *Health Affairs,* Fall.

Schieber, G.J., Poullier, J.-P. and Greenwald, L.M., (1991), ''Health Care Systems in Twenty-Four Countries'', *Health Affairs,* Fall.

Suñol, R., Delgada, R. and Esteban, A., (1991), ''Medical Audit: the Spanish Experience'', *British Medical Journal,* Vol. 303, 16 November.

Young, P. (1990), *European Pharmaceutical Policies,* Adam Smith Institute, London.

112

Chapter 9

THE REFORM OF THE HEALTH SYSTEM IN THE UNITED KINGDOM

INTRODUCTION

The United Kingdom has had a National Health Service (NHS), supplemented by a small, but growing, private sector, since 1948. The first part of this chapter describes the financing and delivery of health services in the United Kingdom and their growth and performance in recent years.

Although the NHS has been, in many ways, a successful institution, there was a crisis of public confidence in the funding and performance of the system in the late 1980s. Following an internal review, the government published a White Paper which set out "... the most far-reaching reform of the National Health Service in its forty-year history" (*Working for Patients,* 1989). In 1989, the government also announced a thorough reform of the arrangements for providing long-term community care services. This involved both the NHS and the separate, personal social services financed by local authorities (*Caring for People,* 1989).

HEALTH CARE SYSTEM DESCRIBED

The health care system in the United Kingdom is dominated by the National Health Service (NHS) which was established to offer comprehensive health services to all the population, originally free of charge to patients. The NHS is financed mainly out of general taxation. Before 1991, "hospital and community health services" (which include home nursing and ambulance services) were provided in public hospitals and by salaried employees, according to the integrated model (see Chapter 2). Most non-hospital services ("family health services") were, and continue to be, supplied by independent practitioners according to the contract model. A small, but growing, independent health care sector is financed partly by direct payments and partly by private insurance under the reimbursement model.

Chart 9.1 shows some of the main features of the financing and delivery of health care in England in 1989. Broadly similar arrangements existed in Scotland, Wales and Northern Ireland. Health services in those parts of the United Kingdom, however, were, and continue to be, financed and administered separately. At the bottom left of the chart is the population, the majority of whom become patients at least once in any year. At the bottom right are some of the main providers of health services. At the top are the third-party payers, public and private. Flows of services are shown as solid lines and flows of finance as broken lines.

Providers have been separated into: pharmacists or retail chemists, who are independent practitioners; general practitioners, likewise independent; public health services; community health services (such as home nursing, ambulances and health visiting); public hospital services (acute and chronic, including out-patient services); private in-patient services supplied in public hospitals; and private hospital and nursing home services supplied by independent providers. Retail pharmacists and private health providers are shown as multiple, indicating competition between them. Until 1991, the public hospital and community health services were financed and managed by district health authorities in an integrated fashion.

Third-party payers have been divided into the Department of Health which in 1989 funded: regional health authorities for the hospital and community health services; and family practitioner committees for the independent practitioner services. Third-party payers also include competing, private, mainly non-profit, insurers which operate mainly according to the principle of reimbursement of patients.

Although regional health authorities are shown among the third-party financiers and district health authorities among the providers, this introduces a somewhat artificial distinction in their roles. In reality, there is a line management relationship between them and in 1989 both authorities combined financing with managerial responsibilities. Thus, regional health authorities were directly responsible for supplying some regional services, for much capital construction, and for employing senior hospital doctors, as well as for funding district health

Chart 9.1 Primary and secondary medical care in England before the 1989 reforms of the NHS
(Financial figures for 1986/87)

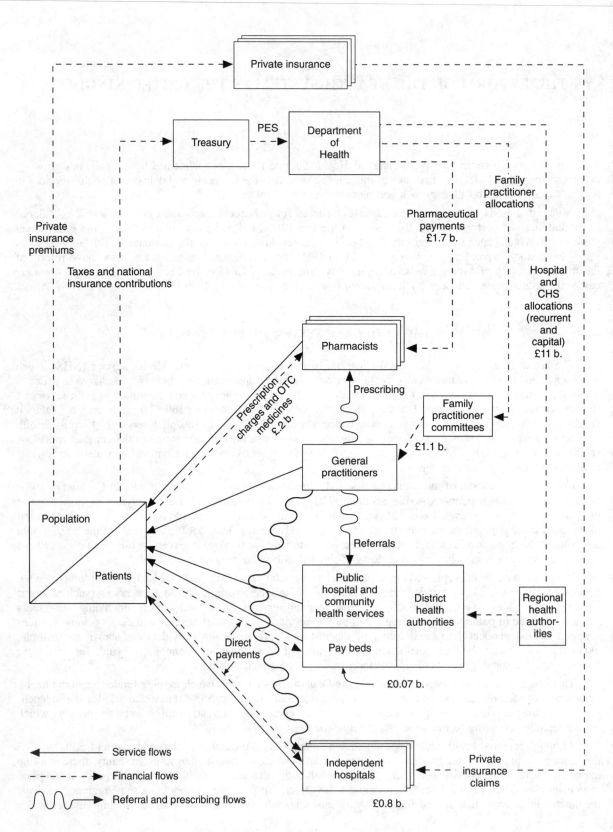

Service flows

Financial flows

Referral and prescribing flows

authorities. District health authorities were responsible for funding hospitals and other units, as well as for the management of the hospital and community health services. This mixing of third-party finance and the management of provision is a characteristic of the integrated model.

General dental and ophthalmic services are also available under the NHS but they have been omitted from the diagram. Also left out of the diagram are public and independent residential and domiciliary personal social services which complement the health services in the area of long-term care.

RELATIONSHIP BETWEEN PATIENTS AND PROVIDERS

General practitioner and pharmaceutical services

People who become sick in the United Kingdom may go to a pharmacist to obtain an over-the-counter medicine. If they wish to consult a doctor they will go usually to the general practitioner (GP) with whom they are registered under the NHS, although they may also visit a hospital accident and emergency department. Most of the population is enrolled with a National Health Service GP, and about 75% of the population's contacts with doctors are handled by GPs. Individuals are free to change their GP, but there is little choice in rural areas; even in urban areas, choice has, until recently, been exercised infrequently, except within group practices or when people change their place of residence. Consultations with general practitioners are free of charge.

Increasingly, general practitioners are organised in group practices, with supporting staff such as receptionists, one or two nurses and even a practice manager. The status of general practitioners is that of independent contractors under the NHS and, in many respects, they operate like small businesses. GPs also act as gatekeepers for most specialist and hospital services.

General practitioners enjoy almost complete clinical autonomy, which includes the freedom: to prescribe, without budgetary restrictions; to refer patients, or pathology specimens, to hospitals for diagnostic tests; and to refer patients to specialists for consultations in hospital out-patient departments. Prescribing and referral rates vary widely between GPs.

If the patient receives a prescription from the GP, it can be taken to the pharmacist. In rural areas, however, doctors dispense drugs themselves. The flat-rate prescription charge was £3.05 in 1990. Many patients are exempt from charges. Those who are not exempt may purchase a "season ticket" (which cost £43.50 per year in 1990) which exempts them from further prescription charges.

Hospital and community health services

The general practitioner may refer a patient whom he or she considers requires specialised diagnosis or treatment, to an NHS hospital or clinic for an out-patient appointment with a specialist or for immediate admission to a bed. Except in cases of emergency, patients often wait a few weeks or even months for an out-patient appointment under the NHS.

The specialist may refer the patient back to the general practitioner, ask the patient to return for another out-patient visit, admit the patient to a bed, or, in the case of elective surgery, put the patient on a waiting list for admission. Later, patients may be referred to the community health services which are linked to the hospitals, for example for home nursing. No charges are payable for out-patient or in-patient care under the National Health Service.

Patients who require treatment which is not available at a typical district general hospital may be referred to a more specialised regional hospital – which is often a teaching hospital. Long-term care is provided in geriatric and psychiatric hospitals and units. However, it has been government policy for at least the past two decades to shift the balance of long-term care away from hospitals towards residential and domiciliary care. The NHS has very few nursing homes.

Private health services

Private medical care is a small but growing sector which plays an essentially complementary role to the NHS. It offers choice of doctor, avoidance of queues for elective surgery, and higher standards of comfort and privacy than the NHS. Private health care is often used in conjunction with the National Health Service, even during the same episode of care. For example, a patient might begin by consulting his/her general practitioner under the NHS, be referred to a specialist as NHS patient, elect for private in-patient care with the same specialist (all senior specialists are allowed to treat private patients), and, on discharge, be referred back to the general practitioner, again under the NHS.

All private care is on a fee-for-service basis. About 8% of acute hospital beds in England are private – 6% in independent hospitals and 2% in public hospitals. However, these beds are mainly devoted to elective surgery and the private sector accounts for as much as one in four of some operations, and for half the abortions carried out in England (Higgins, 1988). There is a private nursing home sector which grew sharply in the 1980s backed by increasing take-up of social security benefits designed to cover some or all of the charges.

Personal social services

Those who require long-term care outside hospitals and nursing homes, particularly the frail elderly, the mentally handicapped and some mentally ill persons, may receive residential or domiciliary care which is financed by local authorities. Charges for these services are means-tested. Private residential and domiciliary care is also available. For individuals on low incomes, care in private residential homes can be funded by social security payments. The take-up of such benefits increased sharply during the 1980s.

RELATIONSHIP BETWEEN THE PATIENTS AND THIRD-PARTY PAYERS

The National Health Service accounted for about 88% of health expenditure in Britain in 1989. The NHS is financed by a mixture of general taxation (79% of expenditure), national insurance contributions (16%) and charges to patients and other miscellaneous payments (5%).

In 1988/89 the part of the national insurance contribution earmarked for the National Health Service was set at 0.95% of earnings for the employee, with an upper earnings limit, and at 0.8% of earnings for the employer, without an upper earnings limit. The self-employed paid 1.75 % of their income.

Voluntary expenditure accounted for about 12% of total health expenditure in 1989. About 70% of this was direct spending, including the purchase of over-the-counter medicines, and about 30% was expenditure on private health insurance, mainly for elective surgery.

About 11% of the population is covered by private health insurance, which is supplied mainly by competing, non-profit insurers. The bulk of subscribers are higher-paid employees and the self-employed, a disproportionate number of whom live in the south-east of England. About one-half of the subscribers are in group schemes with premiums paid for by employers. Such premiums are added to taxable income except for those earning less than £8 500 a year, which is below the average wage. Premiums for groups are generally experience-rated. Premiums for individuals are related to age and rise steeply for elderly people. The cover provided is nowhere near as comprehensive as under the NHS. In the main, the benefits are confined to acute, non-emergency hospital care and to consultations with specialists. About 70% of acute private hospital treatment is funded by insurance (Laing, 1991). A growing proportion of policies not only require deductibles or co-insurance but also restrict cover to particular categories of hospital, or only provide in-patient benefits for subscribers placed on an NHS waiting list. Individuals may be refused insurance cover for pre-existing conditions.

The personal social services are funded by local authorities and are financed by a mixture of local and central taxation and by charges to the users of services. As previously indicated, private expenditure on independent nursing and residential homes during the 1980s was increasingly supported by social security support for the residents.

RELATIONSHIP BETWEEN THIRD-PARTY PAYERS AND PROVIDERS

Expenditure on the NHS is decided by the Cabinet during the annual Public Expenditure Survey. Separate settlements are agreed for England, Scotland, Wales and Northern Ireland. The description which follows applies to England. Money is allocated to the Department of Health separately for the family health services and for the hospital and community health services. The latter, which account for about two-thirds of total expenditure, are cash limited. Once an annual budget has been set, which typically assumes some rises in pay and prices over the previous year, some improvements in efficiency and a margin for growth, it cannot, in principle, be revised during the year. For the most part, family health services are not cash-limited and are often described as "demand-led". Expenditure plans are based on forecasts and supplementary allocations may be made during the year because of unexpected changes in volume or prices. Nevertheless, various controls on the price and/or volume of services ensure that expenditure is contained.

General practitioners and pharmaceutical services

General practitioners are independent contractors and are paid an income plus their practice expenses. Some expenses are paid indirectly via fees and allowances and some are paid directly. Their remuneration, as well as their indirect expenses, are paid through capitation payments, fees for service and practice allowances. There are three levels of *capitation payment,* depending on the age of the patient. Services paid by *fees* include night visiting and immunisation. *Practice allowances* are paid for contingencies, such as setting up in practice and seniority. Remaining expenses, such as rent and rates, are paid for directly.

The average remuneration and average indirect expenses are subject to annual recommendation by an independent Doctors' and Dentists' Review Body (DDRB). Although not bound to do so, the government usually accepts the review body's recommendations. The system is designed to pay exactly the intended remuneration and indirect expenses of the *average* GP. If GPs, on average, provide more than the forecast services, fees and allowances are reduced in proportion to meet the intended average remuneration target. If GPs, on average, incur more or less than forecast expenses, however, fees and allowances are increased or reduced to pay actual expenses. Finally, the global remuneration of the family doctor services rises in proportion to increases in the number of GPs, since for each additional doctor an additional average gross income is added to the pool of money which is made available for distribution.

The remuneration to the individual GP can diverge from the average. Doctors who attract above- or below-average numbers of patients, or who provide an above- or below-average number of fee-paid services, will be paid more or less than the average GP. However, GPs who incur above-average costs for those expenses reimbursed indirectly must meet the extra cost themselves. If they incur below-average costs for such expenses they can keep the savings. There are clearly incentives to "beat the average".

Before April 1989, pharmacists – like GPs, independent practitioners – were paid on a "cost plus" basis for their services to the National Health Service. Since then, however, the body which represents pharmacists has each year negotiated a global sum with the Department of Health, out of which pharmacists are paid dispensing fees for prescriptions according to a sliding scale which tapers according to the volume of prescriptions. Pharmacists are also paid 5% of the net ingredient cost of medicines. If the number of prescriptions fails to reach the level forecast by the Department of Health (and on which the fees are calculated), a lump-sum payment brings remuneration up to the intended level.

Drug prices are controlled under a "pharmaceutical price regulation scheme" (PPRS). The Department of Health controls the maximum profits that drug companies are allowed to earn on their sales of medicines to the NHS. It allows companies commercial freedom to set the relative prices of their products, but can refuse rises in prices which would push total profits above a prescribed level. The Department of Health scrutinises the revenue and costs of the companies, and places a ceiling on the proportion of sales revenue which companies are permitted to devote to the marketing and promotion of products.

Hospital and community health services

Before April 1991, hospital and community health services were financed and managed by regional and district health authorities. The Department of Health made allocations to regional health authorities for the running costs and capital costs of the services, and both allocations were cash-limited. The regions made allocations to district health authorities.

Since the mid-1970s, successive governments have been working to improve the geographical equity of spending on hospital and community health services. A "Resource Allocation Working Party" (RAWP) formula was devised, which set target allocations for regional health authorities based on the size, demographic composition and standardized mortality of their populations, with separate allowances for cross-boundary flows of patients, for teaching hospitals and for London. When the RAWP formula was first introduced, actual allocations differed sharply from these targets. However, for most regions actual allocations have gradually been brought to within a few percentage points of their targets (Social Services Committee, 1989). A similar resource allocation process operates between regional and district health authorities, although the inequities at this level are being eliminated more slowly.

Before April 1991, hospitals and community health services received global budgets, set mainly on a historical basis. Typically, budgets provided for additions for expected rises in pay and prices and planned improvements in services, and deductions for planned improvements in efficiency. Until recently, there was relatively little contracting out of services. Since the mid-1980s, however, competitive tendering for domestic, catering and laundry services in hospitals has been required by law.

Doctors in the hospital and community health services are salaried, they can work part-time and they may receive distinction awards. Their remuneration, like that of general practitioners, is subject to annual review by the independent review body, but the government is not bound by its recommendations. Many consultants also earn private fees. An independent review body also makes recommendations on the remuneration of nurses and some other staff. Wages and salaries of remaining hospital staff are set centrally in direct negotiations between representatives of the employers and the staff.

Capital allocations are also influenced by targets established under the RAWP formula. Parts of these allocations are passed to district health authorities for small building projects and for the acquisition of equipment. Parts are retained by regional health authorities for financing large projects. Regions play a key role in planning such projects. Prior to April 1991, capital expenditure was written off on the completion of projects. In other words, there was no subsequent accounting for depreciation or interest.

Private insurers

Traditionally, private insurers have followed the reimbursement principle. They have reimbursed patients for medical bills rather than entered into direct contracts with providers for the provision of services to their beneficiaries. However, in the face of steep rises in costs, direct negotiations between insurers and providers are becoming more common. Typically, the insurers have tried to persuade the providers to limit their charges in return for being included in a "participating list" of hospitals under their policies (Laing *et al.*, 1988). Benefit limits for medical consultants' fees have been in place for many years, and the profession tends to follow these in submitting bills. This means that there is little extra billing. These arrangements resemble "preferred provider" arrangements in the United States and serve to hold down prices rather than volume, which is determined by doctors and their patients. In an attempt to regulate volume, insurers are increasingly scrutinising and analysing claims, as well as making moves towards managed care.

Personal social services

The personal social services financed by local authorities tend to have a mixture of integrated services – for example, with residential homes owned and financed by local authorities – and contracted services – for example, with residential homes owned and operated by the voluntary sector. Private domiciliary and residential care can also be financed by social security payments.

GOVERNMENT PLANNING AND REGULATION

The National Health Service is an administered system, although it allows considerable professional autonomy to doctors and to other health care professionals. General policy-making is centralised in the Department of Health (in England) but the management of services is partly decentralised.

Family practitioners, including general practitioners and pharmacists, are independent and self-managing. Their relationship with the NHS is contractual. Contracts are administered locally (by family practitioner committees in 1989) but general policy and financing decisions are centralised in the Department of Health.

In 1989, hospital and community health services in England were managed by general managers under the supervision of 14 non-elected regional health authorities and 192 district health authorities. Their chairmen were appointed by the Secretary of State for Health. Most day-to-day management decisions in the hospital and community health services were delegated to district health authorities and to unit managers below them. Regional health authorities were responsible for: allocating budgets to districts; strategic planning and monitoring; managing some regional services; holding the contracts of senior doctors; and making major capital expenditure decisions.

The Department of Health retained responsibility for legislation and general policy matters. The Department was also involved in certain strategic management decisions such as:

– Allocating budgets to regional health authorities;
– Negotiating the wages and salaries of non-review body staff;
– Negotiating drug prices through the pharmaceutical price regulation scheme; and

– Approving major capital expenditure decisions and hospital closures.

Since the mid-1970s, regional health authorities have been required to submit formal plans to the Department of Health. In the early 1980s, the planning system was revised and augmented by a system of regional reviews, which put fresh emphasis on the monitoring of recent performance. General management was introduced into the hospital and community health services in the mid-1980s, with performance-related pay for managers. A central principle of management of the hospital and community health services became delegation downwards and accountability upwards.

Until recently, quality assurance has been patchy in the NHS. A long-standing "confidential inquiry" has looked at maternal deaths and, more recently, two confidential inquiries have investigated peri-operative deaths. An independent Health Advisory Service monitors services for the elderly and mentally ill by means of regular visits to districts. A community health council in each district represents the interests of consumers, and procedures exist to deal with complaints.

The independent health care sector is relatively unregulated, although private hospitals, clinics and nursing homes have to be registered with and inspected by district health authorities.

Personal social services are managed mainly by local authorities. Responsibility for central contributions to local government finance rests with the Department of the Environment. The Department of Health is responsible for central government policy.

GROWTH AND PERFORMANCE

To summarise: The United Kingdom has a comprehensive, tax-financed National Health Service with a small, supplementary, independent health care sector. Expenditure on the NHS is decided by the government. The bulk of spending is cash-limited and, for the rest, financial control by central government is fairly tight. Much of NHS care outside hospitals is supplied by independent contractors, but public bodies and salaried employees provide hospital and domiciliary care.

Table 10.1 shows that the share of health expenditure in GDP increased from 4.5% in 1970 to 5.8% in 1980 and to 6.2% in 1990. GDP rose significantly in the 1980s and the stability in the health expenditure share was accompanied by growth in real health expenditure on the National Health Service. However, much of the growth on expenditure went into increases in the relative prices of health service inputs, especially the pay of doctors and nurses whose remuneration was set following the recommendations of independent review bodies.

In volume terms, inputs to family practitioner services grew at about 2.2% a year and inputs to the Hospital and Community Health Services (HCHS) at about 0.7% a year between 1979/80 and 1988/89 (Social Services Committee, 1989). In addition, measured productivity increased in the Hospital and Community Health Services. A cost-weighted index of HCHS activity rose at about 2% a year over the same period (Social Services Committee, 1990). Voluntary health expenditure outside the NHS grew more rapidly than expenditure inside the NHS, increasing from 8 to 12% of total health expenditure between 1980 and 1989.

Health expenditure per capita was about US$ 758 at purchasing power parity exchange rates in 1987. This was 45% greater than that in Spain and 44% less than that in Germany. Judging by regression analysis linking health expenditure per capita with GDP per capita for OECD countries in 1987 (Schieber and Poullier, 1989), total health expenditure per capita was significantly below the level that would be expected for a country with the standard of living of the United Kingdom.

Table 10.2 suggests that the United Kingdom had fewer physicians and fewer acute hospital beds per 1 000 persons than any of the other six countries in this study. It came fifth out of the seven in its rate of consultations with physicians, and fifth in its acute hospital admission rate. It had the second shortest acute length of stay. The United Kingdom ranked sixth out of the seven countries in medicines prescribed per person, according to a careful, comparative study carried out in 1982. All these figures, except those for numbers of physicians, exclude the (small) independent sector. However, independent sector admissions would have added only 6% to the acute admission rate.

In the independent sector, the numbers voluntarily insured increased by over 50% between 1980 and 1989, to about 11% of the population. There were problems with cost-containment, however. The average premium per person covered rose by about 95% in real terms over the same period (Laing, 1991).

Table 10.3 suggests that the United Kingdom has relatively a better health record than might be expected from its relatively low levels of health expenditure and activity. Among the seven countries in this study, the United Kingdom ranked second for perinatal mortality and third for male expectation of life at birth. However, it ranked only sixth for female expectation of life at birth. The United Kingdom had the second most rapid fall in perinatal mortality between 1980 and 1989.

In terms of the public's satisfaction with health services, the international survey reported in Chapter 10 (Blendon *et al.*, 1990) suggested that only 27% of Britons were satisfied with their health care system, compared with 47% of population in the Netherlands, 41% in the then Federal Republic of Germany and 41% in France. However, the British survey was taken in 1988, at a time when the government was carrying out its review of the National Health Service, a period which saw unprecedented discussion about the future of health services.

During the 1980s evidence was accumulating which pointed to large variations in performance between individual hospitals and between general practitioners. For example, hospital referral rates, admission rates, length of stay and unit costs differ widely (Smee and Parsonage, 1990). The government's aim was to raise the standards of performance of all hospitals and GP practices to those of the best.

There was also evidence that, although the services seemed to perform adequately in terms of health outcomes – and the majority of patients treated were "fairly satisfied" or "very satisfied" with the care which they received (Davies, 1989) – there were failures to meet consumers' needs and preferences. The most conspicuous failure was the long waiting lists for elective surgery (Yates, 1987). By 1990 over 900 000 people were on NHS waiting lists in England alone. Although the median waiting time of patients treated was only five weeks, 23% of those still waiting had waited 12 months or more. Less conspicuous, but equally unsatisfactory, were the long waiting times which were sometimes required for appointments with specialists for routine appointments in hospital out-patient departments (National Audit Office, 1991).

Moreover, the quality of hospital out-patient consultations often left much to be desired. The buildings sometimes had a shabby and run-down appearance. On occasions, patients experienced long waiting times in the out-patient department itself, and the typical patient had only about a 60% chance of seeing a consultant rather than a junior doctor on a first appointment. The consultation itself might be brief and impersonal. There was a marked contrast, here, with the British private sector. It has been said that, "...in an NHS out-patients session the patient listens to the doctor, whereas in a private practice, the consultant listens to the patient" (Sir Thomas Holmes Sellors, quoted in Open University, 1985). Such differences should be kept in perspective, however. Individuals with private insurance still made use of the National Health Service for four-fifths of their out-patient appointments and for one-half of their in-patient stays (Day and Klein, 1989).

Conditions were usually better in general practice, where "family doctoring" encouraged continuity of care. Nevertheless, there were complaints about difficulties of access in deprived areas, inadequate appointment systems and the brevity of the consultation. Although the average length of consultations has increased from perhaps five minutes in the 1950s and 1960s to about eight minutes in the 1980s, it remained short when compared with that in other OECD countries (Wilson, 1991).

Several reasons for these shortcomings have been put forward.

First, for good reasons, patients face virtually no charges and, therefore have no incentive to restrain their demand. On the supply side, services are rationed by means of various expenditure caps, including capitation payments for GPs, salary payments for other doctors and block budgets for hospital and community health services. It is the combination of these demand and supply arrangements which foster queues for service.

Second, before the 1989 reforms aimed at encouraging GPs to be more responsive to their patients, there was little effective choice. People were not encouraged to exercise their right to change their general practitioner. In the case of hospital services, block budgets as well as salary payments for doctors meant that "money did not follow the patient". One result was that patient and doctor choice as between different hospitals was not translated into rewards for the more successful hospitals. Good performance might be rewarded by more work, not by more resources (Enthoven, 1985). Poor performance might be rewarded by an easier life, not by loss of income. A long waiting list could be a weapon with which consultants could bargain for more resources from a hospital or a district health authority.

Third, the allocation of services by doctors was more in accordance with perceived clinical need than with felt consumer preferences (O'Higgins, 1989). This was often appropriate, it was the doctor and not the patient who was sovereign. More generally, allocation decisions were dominated by the providers who usually had a vested interest in the results.

Fourth, although tight budgets provided a general climate of rationing, there were few other incentives – apart from exhortation – to search for cost-savings. Prior to the 1980s, hospitals which regularly made cost-savings might find these diverted elsewhere in the system. The prevalence of block budgets and the lack of price signals throughout the system encouraged providers to think of resources – especially those which fell on some other budget holder to whom the patient could be referred – as "free goods". Because there was no subsequent accounting for capital assets after they were acquired, these could also be considered "free goods".

Fifth, a division of management prevailed throughout the hospital services. Doctors had clinical autonomy but were relatively little involved in general management. General managers had some delegated powers within their budgets but had only limited influence with doctors.

Lastly, information about unit costs and outcome was either lacking or underutilised. The prevailing culture of clinical, non-price rationing, and the absence of competition, were not conducive to the production and use of information on benefits and costs.

All too often, these circumstances – particularly the absence of effective choice on the demand side – conspired to make the health service inflexible, paternalistic and, in some ways, unresponsive to patients. Major emergencies tended to elicit prompt and effective care. However, the treatment of minor, non-urgent or intractable illness, especially by specialists, might be delayed, inconvenient and impersonal. And, to judge by the growing evidence on the variability of performance indicators discussed above, the effectiveness of divided hospital management was, at best, patchy.

The personal social services managed by local authorities experienced somewhat similar weaknesses. However, one of the most pressing concerns for the government towards the end of the 1980s in the area of long-term care was the rapid growth of private nursing and residential care funded out of an open-ended social security budget. This not only brought about a crisis of cost-containment, but also conflicted with the government's policy of supporting elderly and handicapped people in their own homes for as long as possible.

BACKGROUND TO THE REFORMS IN THE EIGHTIES

In many ways, the National Health Service was a successful institution before the reforms set out in the 1989 White Paper, *Working for Patients*. The service provided universal access to health care, allocated on the basis of need. It gave income protection to the sick. It employed skilled and conscientious doctors and gave them considerable clinical (and, in the case of GPs, managerial) autonomy. The service was also relatively cheap to provide and to administer. One estimate suggested that, at 6%, administration costs as a percentage of total expenditure were less than one-third those in the United States, at 22% (Himmelstein and Woolhandler, 1986). Furthermore, such indicators of health outcome as existed suggested that the United Kingdom's health services performed adequately.

However, the National Health Service had always suffered from a number of problems, some of which intensified during the 1980s. One was persistent controversy over the level of spending. Successive conservative governments during the 1980s were determined that public expenditure should take a declining share of national income. However, real spending on health was actually increased by the government during the 1980s. Nevertheless, the government's critics argued that the real growth of the hospital and community health services budget was not enough to match growing demand from: demographic change, estimated to add 1% per annum to "need"; from new, costly medical techniques; and from planned improvements in services (Social Services Committee, 1986; Robinson and Judge, 1987). The government responded to these criticisms by pointing to steady improvements in hospital productivity. Their argument was that performance should be judged, not by the level of inputs to the NHS, but by its outputs.

Nevertheless, the government came under increasing pressure concerning the level of spending on the National Health Service prior to its setting up of the internal Review in January 1988. The government approached the Review with the conviction that the way to meet growing demand was not to inject more money into the health service, but to raise its productivity further by reforming the way in which the service was both organised and managed (*Working for Patients*, 1989).

REFORMS TO THE NHS IN THE EIGHTIES

Reforms prior to the 1988/89 Review of the NHS

Prior to the major reform announced in January 1988, the government introduced a number of lesser but important reforms to the National Health Service during the 1980s.

In 1982, the government abolished a whole tier of health authorities – the area health authorities – which had been created as a result of a previous reorganisation in 1974. Systematic, annual reviews of the performance of regional and district health authorities were also introduced in 1982, and work began on the construction of a package of performance indicators for regions, districts and units which laid particular stress on measures of their activity and unit costs. Similar reviews were introduced for family practitioner committees in 1985.

In 1983, the government commissioned Sir Roy Griffiths – managing director of the Sainsbury's supermarket chain – to carry out a review of the management of the NHS. Griffiths diagnosed a state of "institutionalised stagnation" in the NHS: "if Florence Nightingale were carrying her lamp through the corridors of the NHS she would almost certainly be searching for the people in charge" (Griffiths, 1983). Griffiths recommended that the existing system of consensus management should be replaced by a system of general management throughout the health service, with supervisory and management boards based in the Department of Health. General managers could be brought in from outside the health service, and their pay should be related to performance.

Also in 1983, district health authorities were obliged to introduce competitive tendering for cleaning, laundry and catering services in the hospital and community health service. Private firms were encouraged to compete against the existing services which relied on directly employed staff.

Between 1980 and 1985, a review of NHS information requirements was carried out. This led to major revisions to the new systems for collecting statistics and new data began to be available from 1987/88. From the mid-1980s, experiments were started in a few large hospitals under the "resource management initiative". The aim was to tackle the problem of divided hospital management and to improve the quality of information on which decisions could be made.

In 1984, a limited list for drugs was introduced the main effect of which was to remove a large number of household medicines from payment under the NHS.

In 1987, following public consultation, the government published a White Paper on the then family practitioner services (*Promoting Better Health,* 1987). One of the main purposes of the White Paper was to propose ways in which general practitioners could be encouraged to be more responsive to their patients. This was to be done by tightening their conditions of service and by introducing more competition between doctors for patients. More competition would be achieved by increasing the capitation element in general practitioners' remuneration, by making it easier for patients to change doctors and by requiring doctors to provide more information on the services which they offered, such as surgery opening hours.

The White Paper also contained proposals to: encourage the supply of health promotion and preventive services by paying general practitioners for reaching targets on child immunisation and cervical screening; strengthen primary health care teams by allowing doctors to take on more staff; and encourage substitution of GP care for hospital care by, for example, paying fees to GPs for carrying out minor surgery. These proposals were not well received by general practitioners. Nevertheless, the Department of Health introduced a new contract in 1990 (Health Department of Great Britain, 1989).

The 1988/89 Review of the NHS

The 1988/89 Review of the NHS arose out of a crisis of public confidence in the funding and performance of the health service. Day and Klein (1989) have written of the situation in 1987: "Never before in the history of the NHS had there been such a public demonstration of concern, involving all the authoritative figures in the health care policy arena". The government responded by setting up an internal Review in January 1988, chaired by the then Prime Minister Margaret Thatcher. The review was accompanied by an unprecedented public debate about the funding and organisation of the NHS (Brazier *et al.,* 1988; Goldsmith and Willetts, 1988; the Institute of Health Services Management, 1988; Kings Fund Institute, 1988; Robinson, 1988). Some of the key ideas adopted in the reforms had been put forward earlier by Maynard (1986) and Enthoven (1985).

The White Paper, *Working for Patients* (1989), which resulted from the Review, contained proposals which were designed to build on the strengths of the NHS and to tackle its weaknesses. No changes were proposed in the sources of finance of the NHS, and hence in the demand from patients. The White Paper envisaged that services would still be funded out of general taxation and would be mainly free of charge to the patient. However, there was to be a separation of the purchasing and provision of hospital services, mediated by contracts. District health authorities would become, in the main, purchasers of hospital services. Some general practitioners would be able to volunteer to have transferred to them part of the hospital budget and to become purchasers. Meanwhile, well-managed public hospitals would be freed from the control of district health authorities and would be allowed to become "self-governing".

In effect, the changes involved a move away from the integrated model towards a form of contract model for the hospital services, together with a form of managed competition on the supply side. The family health services were to be put under the supervision of the regional health authorities. All these proposals were designed to improve the flexibility and efficiency of the NHS, without reducing its equity. Whereas the means by which

Chart 9.2 **The British health care system after the 1989 reforms**

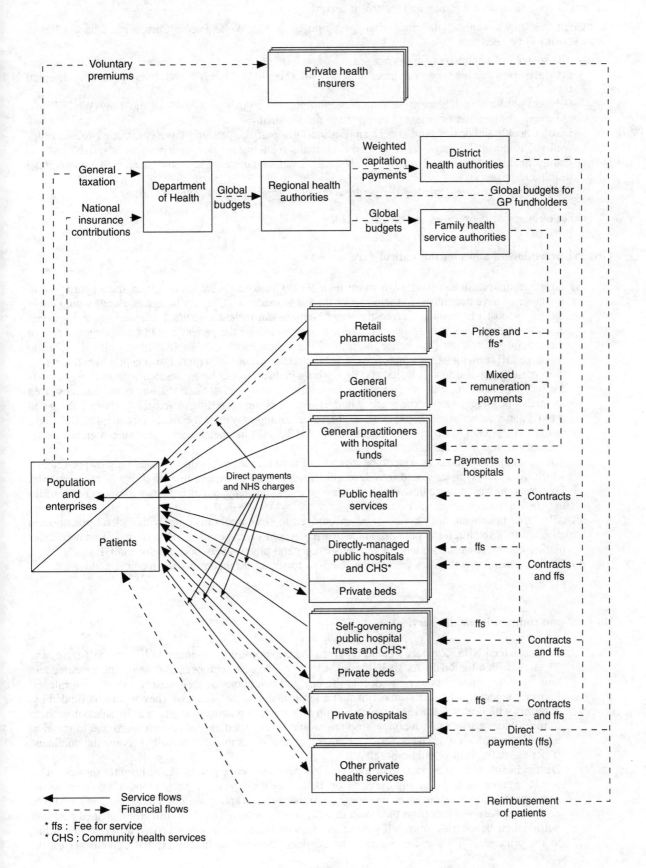

Service flows
Financial flows

* ffs : Fee for service
* CHS : Community health services

health services were delivered would involve managed markets, the ends would continue to include payment for services according to ability to pay and treatment according to need.

Chart 9.2 shows some of the main changes proposed in the White Paper. Comparing Chart 9.2 with Chart 9.1, it can be seen that:

- The sources of finance remain unchanged;
- Providers now include general practitioners with (hospital) ''funds'' and ''self-governing hospital trusts'';
- GPs and public hospitals are now shown as multiple, the former as a result of the 1987 White Paper, indicating competition or potential competition among them;
- District health authorities now appear among the third-party payers and have contractual relationships with public hospitals (they may also have contractual relationships with independent hospitals);
- Family health authorities (formerly family practitioner committees) are now accountable to regional health authorities;
- GPs who hold hospital ''funds'' derive these directly from regional health authorities.

Other elements of the reforms are described below.

General practitioners and pharmaceutical care

i) Large group practices (those with more than 9 000 patients) were to be given the opportunity to volunteer to have transferred to them part of the funds made available for hospitals. Funds would cover the likely cost of: hospital diagnostic tests; hospital out-patient consultations; and some in-patient elective surgery. This was designed to allow money to follow the patient and to strengthen the arm of the general practitioner (and hence the arm of the patient) with the hospital. It was also designed to make the GP conscious of hospital costs. GP fundholders would be required to accept a firm budget for their prescribing of drugs. Hospital and prescribing budgets would be aggregated with existing budgets for staff costs and improvements to practice premises. Savings under one heading could be transferred to another heading. Initially, the practice budgets would be set according to actual (past) prescribing and referral patterns, but eventually they would be set according to weighted capitation principles. If the cost falling on the budget of any one patient exceeded £5 000 in one financial year, the regional health authority would meet the extra cost.

ii) The remaining GP practices were to be given indicative prescribing budgets, based on past prescribing, which, for the first time, would introduce guidelines related to expenditure on drugs in each practice. The intention was to place downward pressure on expenditure by enhancing consciousness of prescribing costs among general practitioners.

iii) All district health authorities were to be encouraged to enter into a dialogue with general practitioners about their hospital referral patterns, since districts would be responsible, in consultation with GPs, for placing contracts with hospitals for referrals by general practitioners not paid for via GP funds.

iv) Finally, general practitioners were to be required to set up arrangements for medical audit with their peers.

Hospital and community health services

i) Well-managed NHS hospitals were to be given the opportunity to volunteer to become self-governing ''trusts'' within the NHS. As such, they would be expected to compete, and would be given certain new freedoms such as powers to: decide the pay and conditions of their staff; accumulate surpluses; borrow, subject to an overall annual financial limit; and dispose of assets. They would be funded by: contracts with health authorities; contracts with GPs holding practice budgets; and by sales of services to the private sector. Self-governing hospitals would be expected to service their loans and to make an agreed return on capital. The government envisaged that trusts might eventually become the dominant, if not the only, form of public hospital.

ii) District health authorities were to be expected to operate as active purchasers of hospital services. This would involve them in buying services on behalf of their resident populations after carrying out assessments of health care needs, mounting consumer surveys and consulting their GPs. They would be able to purchase services from their own directly managed hospitals, from directly managed hospitals outside their boundaries, from self-governing trusts and from independent private hospitals, according to the principles of value for money. The services required, including explicit agreements on the quality of services required from the main local supplier, and their prices, would be specified explicitly in contracts. Since not all needs could be foreseen, there would be provision for extra contractual referrals. Districts would be expected to purchase some services, such as accident and emergency services, locally. Such services should be available immediately for any patient who needed them, irrespective of their district of residence.

iii) District health authorities (after a transition period) were to be funded for their resident populations, according to a weighted capitation formula, rather than for the services provided within their boundaries. They would still be cash-limited.

iv) Hospitals were to be encouraged to compete, meanwhile, for the contracts with districts. These might be block contracts initially, but might increasingly become cost and volume or cost per case contracts. The hospitals should set prices for individual services based on cost and a 6% return on capital. There should be no cross-subsidisation between individual services. There was to be a provision for arbitration in case of contractual disputes. Since "money would follow the patient", hospitals would be given new incentives to satisfy patients and to minimise costs.

v) All NHS hospitals were to be given the freedom to generate income by marketing services to private individuals and enterprises, including better hotel care to patients.

vi) For the first time in the history of the NHS, the cost of existing capital was to be recognised by: valuing the stock; charging interest and depreciation: including capital charges in the prices of contracts; and adding to the recurrent funding of district health authorities to meet these charges. This would ensure that the right prices were set within the NHS and that there would be "a level playing field" with the private sector. In other words, capital would no longer be a "free" good.

vii) At the same time, better information on the quality of services was to be required. Doctors would be obliged to engage in medical audit by their peer groups within hospitals. Although the detailed results would be confidential, the general results should be available to managers and should be published widely.

viii) In addition, the financial audit of the NHS would be transferred from the Health Department to the independent Audit Commission. The Commission's remit would include investigation of the value for money of services.

ix) The contracts of hospital consultants were to be revised. There would be clear job descriptions, revised annually. District health authority managers were to be involved in the appointment of consultants, although their contracts would continue to be held by regional health authorities. The system of distinction awards was to be amended. Senior doctors' commitment to management and the development of services would be added criteria for the lowest "C" award, general managers would be represented on the committees making the "C" awards, and the awards would be made reviewable after five years.

x) Finally, tax relief was to be granted for private health insurance premiums purchased by or on behalf of elderly people.

Timetable for implementation

The White Paper set out an ambitious timetable for the implementation of the reforms, as follows:

- During 1989, the first hospitals to become self-governing were to be identified, regulations were to be introduced to make it easier for patients to change their general practitioners, districts were to begin to agree job descriptions with their consultants, the new framework for medical audit was to be implemented, preparations for introducing indicative drug budgets for GPs were to begin and the Audit Commission was to start its work on the NHS.
- During 1990, these changes were to gain momentum, and regional and district health authorities, as well as family practitioner committees, were to be reorganised.
- During 1991, the first NHS hospital trusts were to be set up, the first GP fundholders were to be established, indicative drug budgets were to be implemented and districts were to begin paying directly for the work which they carried out for one another.

Reform of long-term community care

In November 1989, following a report by Sir Roy Griffiths (1988), the government announced proposals for the reform of long-term community care services for the elderly, the mentally and physically handicapped and the mentally ill. Involving all the relevant public and independent agencies – including local authority personal social services, the NHS, and the social security services – , the reforms introduced a new funding structure for those who seek public support for residential and nursing home care (*Caring for People,* 1989). Residents of homes in the independent sector are to receive social security benefits on the same basis as people in their own homes, instead of the current, special higher rates of benefit. Local authorities will take over responsibility for financial support for residents of these homes, over and above the general social security entitlements. In effect, part of the open-ended social security budget is to be taken over by local authorities, and is likely to be capped.

Local authorities, in collaboration with other agencies, are to become responsible for assessing individuals' needs, designing care arrangements and securing their delivery within available resources. They are to be encouraged to become "enabling agencies" making maximum use of the independent sector. The government's main aims in reforming long-term community care include the promotion of domiciliary, day and respite services to enable people to live in their own homes wherever appropriate, and the development of more practical support for informal carers. Other key objectives include: improved assessment of need; more reliance on care managers; improved co-ordination between care agencies; promotion of the mixed economy of care; and removal of the incentives that higher rates of social security payments gave towards residential care. Originally, it was the government's intention that the reforms should take effect from the beginning of April 1991. In July 1990, however, the government announced that the changes would be phased in between 1991 and 1993. It was reported that this was because of concern about the likely upward pressure on the new, local authority community charge or poll tax (*Financial Times,* 10th July 1990).

Preliminary assessment of the reforms

There were three major reforms to the health and personal social services of the United Kingdom in prospect at the end of the 1980s involving: remuneration of general practitioners; the financing and organisation of the National Health Service; and community care. It is possible to identify at least four common threads running through the reforms:

- Third-party payers were to be funded by global budgets (to be mainly set according to weighted capitation principles);
- Third-party payers were to behave as active purchasers;
- Providers were to be given more autonomy and encouraged to compete for fixed public funds;
- Payer/provider relationships were to be mediated by contracts, with money following the patient.

These reforms provoked much debate with the following issues being the subject of particular scrutiny.

Although consumers were to be given more effective choice between GPs and, through GP fundholders, between hospitals, they were not to be given choice among district health authorities. This led to questions about whether the right incentives were in place for districts to act in the best interest of consumers. Indeed, in fixing contracts with hospitals, they might actually reduce GP and consumer choice. However, districts were required to consult GPs and to carry out surveys of consumer opinion before placing contracts.

In the case of GP fundholders, questions were raised about risk selection among patients. The concern was that there would be considerable incentives for general practitioner fundholders to "skim the cream" by selecting healthier patients for their lists. Although general practitioners already faced such incentives in their existing remuneration system, fundholding status strengthened the incentives to "skim". This was because some hospital services were no longer "free" goods and surplus funds could be diverted to the practices themselves. However, it seemed likely that weighted capitation payments and regulations could be devised to counteract tendencies towards "skimming".

Considerable discussion also surrounded the issue of how efficiently and fairly provider markets would work in the reformed National Health Service.

- Concern was expressed that, given the difficulty of measuring both health outcome and the quality of care, competition would lead to volume for money but not value for money. For example, difficult cases might be under-served or patients asked to travel long distances to reduce the cost of care. This risk was clearly recognised, and, accordingly, emphasis was laid on developing adequate measures of quality in the placing of contracts. In addition, guidance was given on the need for both district and family health service authorities to conduct surveys of consumer satisfaction.
- A different concern was that, with government on both sides of the market, competition would not be allowed to work properly. For example, the government might be tempted to intervene to block public hospital closures precipitated by competition. However, the government stated that it recognised that there were likely to be losers as well as gainers from the competitive process (MacLachlan, 1991).

- The government's hope was that the reforms would reduce the pressure for extra spending on the National Health Service. However, the government was also aware that, in some respects, there would be extra pressure on costs. The reforms called for considerable investment in information and management systems to support the internal market. For example, some large hospitals faced the need to negotiate 60 or 70 contracts to replace what had previously been one allocation. Worries were also expressed that the freedom granted to self-governing hospital trusts to set pay and conditions for their staff would lead to upward pressures on pay (which accounts for about 70% of running costs) throughout the hospital service. In the case of junior hospital doctors, the government decided to maintain national pay scales for self-governing trusts. Some thought that the greater transparency in resource allocation decisions would be a further source of pressure on public expenditure.

- There were risks that either monopsony or monopoly power might be abused in the new market. The risk of abuse of monopoly power seemed particularly great, with some hospitals dominating their local catchment areas outside large cities and fragmentation of purchasing power between districts and GP fundholders. However, such risks were countered by regulations which required: hospitals to charge their services at cost (including a fixed return on capital); and prices and contracts to be published openly (thereby encouraging "yardstick" competition). Also, there was early formation of buying consortia among some districts and GP fundholders. Measurement of hospital concentration suggested that hospital markets would be tolerably competitive (Robinson, 1991).

- The speed at which the reforms were carried out gave rise to controversy. Critics argued that changes of such a size and complexity were unpredictable in their effects and should have been the subject of pilot studies. However, formal piloting would have greatly extended the timetable for implementation of the reforms. The formation of hospital trusts and GP fundholding practices was voluntary and evolutionary, allowing for "learning by doing". Moreover, the government was able to build into the implementation process a series of "development projects" on a number of important issues – for example, purchasing and contracting – and, later, a series of "localities projects", which involved demonstrations in seven districts of the full package of reforms. These assisted in the identification of difficulties and in the diffusion of management solutions.

- Finally, concern was expressed that the split of purchasing authority in the area of long-term care between districts and local authorities might impede the transfer of patients out of long-term hospitals and would discourage integration of care. This, however, was not a new problem and measures have been taken to require health authorities and family health services authorities to draw up and publish community care plans which will be compatible with those of their matching local authorities.

Implementation of the reforms and early results

Implementation of reforms to the NHS went ahead as planned. A new contract for general practitioners was introduced in 1990. In April 1991, 57 NHS hospitals and units became self-governing trusts, 306 GP practices became fundholders, all districts had separated their purchasing and providing functions and most had finalised contracts with hospital providers. A second wave of 99 trusts and GP fundholders joined the initial group in April 1992. Over one million NHS assets had been valued so that prices could include capital charges. On average these added 17% to recurrent costs. For the most part, new job plans had also been agreed with consultants.

The government indicated that it wanted most of the existing patient flows to be maintained in the first year of contracting (1991/92). The aim was to achieve a "smooth take-off" as purchasers and providers became used to working with the new system. Indeed, there were signs that a learning process was required. For example, in any of the proposed contracts signed between districts and providers for the first year were block contracts. Where prices were fixed for individual services, major variations in the prices of similar services were reported, partly because of differences in accountancy practices.

In July 1991, the government announced a timetable for putting the funding of regional and district health authorities on a weighted capitation basis. It also announced that health authorities would be free from April 1992 to switch contracts to different hospitals if this would be in the interest of patients.

By the end of 1991, evidence was already accumulating that suggested that the reforms were beginning to alter the culture of the NHS.

The new contract for GPs quickly produced significant changes in behaviour and the provision of a wider range of services by GPs. There was an immediate surge of activity in response to the new performance-related parts of the contract, involving in particular: vaccination and immunisation for children; health promotion clinics; and minor surgery. This led to an overpayment, in relation to the intended net target income for the average GP, of about 15% in 1990/91. In November 1991, it was announced that about one-third of this overpayment would be exempted from the normal arrangements to "claw back" excess payments in subsequent years. Meanwhile, the extra services seem to have been appreciated by patients. A survey revealed that three out of ten patients had noticed an improvement in the service they received from their GP since the introduction of the new contract.

GP fundholding was also showing conspicuous results. Fundholders were finding that their new purchasing power had transformed their bargaining position with hospitals. Many had drawn up agreements with hospitals spelling out quality standards for their patients on matters such as the way they were treated by hospital staff, and the information on their treatment which was fed back to the practice. Others had persuaded specialists to hold clinics on the GPs premises to suit the convenience of their patients. There were signs that fundholders had won more influence over hospital specialists in six months than lay managers had gained in several decades. There was, however, immediate controversy about "two-tier care" and the government introduced regulations discouraging hospitals from discriminating between the patients of GP fundholders and the patients of other GPs.

At the same time, the holding of hospital budgets was encouraging a new consciousness about hospital costs among fundholders. Fundholders had begun to shop around for hospital care for their patients and to question the necessity for some hospital work, such as repeated visits by their patients to out-patients clinics.

Fundholding seemed to have been a success with most GPs who had participated in the scheme. A survey carried out about halfway through 1991 suggested that: 89% of fundholders would continue into a second year; 11% were undecided; and not a single fundholder intended to withdraw from the scheme.

The setting up of DHAs as purchasers had stimulated them to focus in a new way on the needs of their resident populations and on the possibilities for securing cost-effective care from alternative hospital providers. Many DHAs had specified quality standards for their patients in their contracts. Many had conducted surveys of the referral preferences of GPs and the satisfaction of patients.

There was less to report about responses on the supply side, because of the moratorium on changes in DHA contracts in the first year. However, there was every sign that as DHAs prepared to switch some of their contracts in April 1992, providers were working to improve their competitiveness. Also, purchasing, combined with capital charges, seemed to have brought a new air of realism into the investment programme. The case for some large new hospitals, then in the pipeline, was suddenly found to be wanting. The case for certain other investments – in day surgery facilities, for example – suddenly became overwhelming.

There was concern that because there were high prices and probably spare capacity in the London area, the new NHS market would threaten the viability of some hospital providers, including some large teaching hospitals, there. The government set up an enquiry into the particular problems of London in October 1991 and suspended temporarily the setting up of further trusts in the capital. This might be regarded as an example of putting "management" into the "managed market". In October 1992, the Report requested recommended that ten hospitals be phased out, including a few teaching hospitals.

There were signs that the new "self-governing" trusts were using their greater managerial freedoms to improve the quality and efficiency of their services. Several had announced reductions in in-patient length of stay, increases in activity and reductions in waiting times. Several had conducted their own surveys of consumers' views and satisfaction. There had been concern that some trusts would face financial difficulties by the end of the first year but most were forecasting that they would achieve financial balance.

Finally, improved procedures for medical audit had been welcomed by the medical and nursing professions and systematic peer-group scrutiny of clinical practice both by nurses and doctors had become widely established.

CONCLUSION

The early results provide some encouragement that the reforms have begun to achieve their intended effects. In particular, GP fundholders have shown themselves to be capable of improving the responsiveness of hospital services for their patients. This tackles head on what was, probably, the outstanding weakness of the NHS. It remained to be seen, however, whether a similar effect can be extended to all patients and whether the problem of patient selection can be avoided in the longer term.

More generally, these early results leave unanswered most of the questions raised in the last section. The separation of purchasers and providers in the National Health Service requires the learning of new roles and is likely to lead to a long process of consequential adjustments to behaviour and to services. The creation of GP fundholders and self-governing trusts will be voluntary and evolutionary, and the process might be halted or reversed by a future government. For these reasons, no full assessment of the 1991 reforms to the NHS could be made at the time this report was completed.

References

Blendon, R.J., Leitman, R., Morrison, I. et Donelan, K. (1990), "Satisfaction with health systems in ten nations", *Health Affairs,* Summer.

Brazier, J., Hutton, J. and Jeavons, R. (1988), *Reforming the UK Health Care System.* Centre for Health Economics, Health Economics Consortium, 1988 Discussion paper 47. York, University of York.

Caring for People (1989), *Community Care in the Next Decade and Beyond,* HMSO, November.

Day, P. and Klein, R. (1989), "The Politics of Modernisation: Britain's National Health Service in the 1980s", *The Milbank Quarterly,* Vol. 67, No. 1.

Davies, P. (1989), "The NHS Goes to the Opinion Polls", *The Health Service Journal,* 22 June.

Enthoven, A.C. (1985), *Reflections on the Management of the National Health Service,* Nuffield Provincial Hospitals Trust.

Goldsmith, M. and Willetts, D. (1988), *Managed Health Care,* Centre for Policy Studies, London.

The Government's Expenditure Plans, 1989-90 to 1991-92 (1989), Department of Health, Cm 614, HMSO, London.

Griffiths, R. (1983), *Report of the NHS Management Enquiry,* Department of Health and Social Security, London.

Griffiths, R. (1988), *Community Care: Agenda for Action,* HMSO, London.

Harrison, A. (1990), "Cost-Containment in the NHS, 1979-1990", in *Health Care UK, 1990,* Policy Journals.

Health Department of Great Britain (1989), *General Practice in the National Health Service: the 1990 Contract,* August, London.

Higgins J. (1988), *The Business of Medicine: Private Health Care in Britain,* Macmillan.

Himmelstein, D.U. and Woolhandler, S. (1986), "Cost without benefit: Administrative waste in U.S. health care", *New England Journal of Medicine,* 314(7).

Institute of Health Services Management (1988), *Working Party on Alternative Delivery and Funding of Health Service, Final Report,* London.

King's Fund Institute (1988), *Health Finance, Assessing the Options,* London.

Laing, W., (1991), *Laing's Review of Private Healthcare 1990-91,* Laing and Buisson, London.

Laing, W., Bricknell, B., Forman, R. and Saldana, N. (1988), *Keeping the Lid on Costs? Essays on private health insurance and cost-containment in Britain,* Institute of Economic Affairs, Health Unit, London.

MacLachlan, R. (1991), "Message to the troops on the eve of battle", *The Health Service Journal,* 28 March.

Maynard, A. (1986), "Performance Incentives in General Practice", in *Health, Education and General Practice,* Teeling Smith, G. (ed.), Office of Health Economics, London.

National Audit Office (1991), *NHS Out-patient Services,* HMSO, London, February.

O'Higgins, M. (1989), "Dilemmas of NHS", in Collard, D. (ed.), *Fiscal Policy,* Gower, London.

Open University (1985), *Caring for Health: Dilemmas and Prospects,* Open University Press.

Promoting Better Health (1987), The Government's Programme for Improving Primary Health Care, HMSO, London.

Robinson, R. (1988), *Efficiency and the NHS: A Case for Internal Markets.* The IEA Health Unit, London.

Robinson, R. (1991), "Who's playing monopoly?", *The Health Service Journal,* 28 March.

Robinson, R. and Judge, K. (1987), *Public Expenditure and the NHS: Trends and Prospects,* King's Fund Institute, London.

Schieber, G. and Poullier, J.-P. (1989), "International Health Care Expenditure Trends: 1987", *Health Affairs,* Fall.

Smee, C. and Parsonage, M. (1990), "Reform of the United Kingdom National Health Service: an Economic Perspective", paper prepared for the Second World Congress on Health Economics, University of Zurich, September.

Social Services Committee (1986), *Public Expenditure and the Social Services,* House of Commons, Session 1985-86, HC387, HMSO, London.

Social Services Committee (1989), *Resourcing the National Health Service: The Government's Plans for the Future of the National Health Service,* House of Commons, Session 1988-89, July (214 - III), HMSO, London.

Social Services Committee (1990), *Public Expenditure on Health Matters,* House of Commons, Session 1989-90: 484, June, HMSO, London.

Wilson, A. (1991), "Consultation length in general practice: a review", *British Journal of General Practice,* March.

Working for Patients (1989), HMSO, London.

Yates, J. (1987), *Why Are We Waiting?,* Oxford University Press.

Chapter 10

GROWTH AND PERFORMANCE OF
THE SEVEN HEALTH CARE SYSTEMS

The purpose of this chapter is to compare the growth and performance of the health care systems in the seven countries with a view to shedding further light on the circumstances which gave rise to the reforms and, where possible, on their effects. The data are derived from a variety of sources, including the OECD health data base, and build on the evidence and analysis contained in an earlier OECD publication, *Financing and Delivering Health Care* (OECD, 1987). It should be borne in mind that strict definitional consistency of data on health, health care activity and health care expenses across these countries has not yet been achieved.

LEVEL AND GROWTH OF HEALTH EXPENDITURE

Table 10.1 shows aggregate data on health expenditure in the seven countries. Culyer (1989) has reviewed the econometric literature on the determinants of health expenditure across countries. His findings suggest that health expenditure per capita and the proportion of income spent on health are both greater the higher is GDP per capita. Health expenditure is also lower than might be expected in countries with centralised control of health care budgets. Subsequent econometric analysis by Gerdtham *et al.* (1990) has suggested five variables which contribute significantly to an explanation of differences in per capita health expenditures across OECD countries: per capita GDP, with an expenditure elasticity of 1.06; the age dependency ratio, with an expenditure elasticity of 0.22; the proportion of public financing to total financing, with an expenditure elasticity of –0.23; the ratio of in-patient health care expenditure to total health care expenditure, with an expenditure elasticity of 0.37; and the presence of global budgeting in hospitals, which is associated, on average, with a 13% reduction in health expenditure, other things being equal.

The evidence presented in Table 10.1 is consistent with these findings. Looking first at the data for 1990 in column 1, most of the variation recorded there in health expenditure per capita is explained by a regression line which links per capita health expenditure with per capita GDP (Schieber and Poullier, 1989). Allowing for a possible underestimation of health expenditure in Belgium and Germany, per capita health expenditure would lay above the regression line for the first four countries in the table. These relied mainly on the reimbursement and contract models and had only adopted global budgets for some or all hospitals in the mid-1980s. The United Kingdom, which had relied mainly on central tax funding and had had global budgeting in hospitals for four decades, lay sharply below the line.

Turning to the time series evidence in columns 2-7, what is most striking is the fact that all seven countries reduced sharply the rate of growth of their health expenditure in relation to GDP between 1980 and 1990 compared with the decade between 1970 and 1980. Looking more closely at the period between 1980 and 1990, the countries can be put into three groups. The two countries which still relied to some extent on the reimbursement model, and which had only partially adopted global budgets during the 1980s, Belgium and France, saw an average rise in their health expenditure shares of 14% compared with an average rise of 17% in their real, per capita GDPs, except for the years 1989 and 1990. The two countries which relied mainly on the contract model, and which had adopted global budgets more comprehensively, Germany and the Netherlands, saw virtually no change in their health expenditure shares, despite an average rise of 14% in real, per capita GDPs. The three countries which relied mainly on the integrated model, and which had operated hospital global budgets for many years, Ireland, Spain and the United Kingdom, saw widely differing changes in their health expenditure shares. Spain was still building up services from a low base but at a modest rate given rapid growth in its GDP. Ireland continued to cut back services from a high base despite vigorous economic recovery. The United Kingdom

Table 10.1. Health expenditure and health expenditure shares of GDP

	Health expenditure per capita at purchasing power parity	Health expenditure as a percentage share of GDP			Percentage change in health expenditure share		Percentage change in GDP per capita at constant prices
	1990	1970	1980	1990	1970-80	1980-90	1980-90
Belgium	1 227	4.1*	6.6	7.6	61*	15	20
France	1 532	5.8	7.6	8.8	31	16	18
Germany	1 487	5.9	8.4	8.1	42	–4	20
Ireland	819	5.6*	9.6	7.5	71*	–22	39
Netherlands	1 287	6.0	8.0	8.0	33	0	14
Spain	777	3.7	5.6	6.5	51	18	28
United Kingdom	974	4.5	5.8	6.2	29	7	28

* The 1970 level may be slightly underestimated, owing to a break in the series, and the change 1970-1980 consequently overstated.
Source: OECD Health Systems: Facts and Trends, 1993, Paris.

maintained a constant health expenditure share despite strong growth in its economy. On average, this group saw virtually no change in its health expenditure share, despite a rise of 24% in real, per capita GDP.

Given the expected positive association between health expenditure shares and per capita GDP, this evidence suggests that the countries with mainly integrated systems exercised stronger cost containment than those with contract systems. In turn, countries with contract systems exercised stronger cost containment than those with continuing attachment to the reimbursement model and which had only partially adopted global budgets.

HEALTH CARE RESOURCES AND ACTIVITY

Table 10.2 presents some aggregate, cross-sectional data from the OECD health data base, and other sources, on physician numbers and activity and acute hospital beds and activity in an attempt to identify effects due to differences in payment systems. Time series on such variables are too patchy to be presented here. Bearing in mind that complete definitional consistency of the data has yet to be attained, the figures are nonetheless worth examining for the variations across countries which they reveal. The first four columns provide evidence that the first three countries – all of which allow free choice of primary care physician for each service and pay primary care physicians by fee for service – have higher consultation rates, longer consultation times and higher prescribing rates than the Netherlands, Spain and the United Kingdom, which pay most physicians by capitation or salary. There is no sign that variations in the number of doctors per capita play a role in these differences. Time series evidence supports the conclusion that, compared with capitation payments, fee for service encourages consultations. For example, it was reported that consultation rates with GPs by public patients in Ireland fell by about a fifth in the year which followed the switch, in March 1989, from fee-for-service to capitation payments.

Turning to the last three columns of Table 10.2, which deal with acute hospitals, large differences exist between the seven countries in number of acute beds per thousand. There are some signs that these differences may be associated with health expenditure per capita and public ownership. Ireland, Spain and the United Kingdom, with a high proportion of public beds, have fewer acute beds per thousand than Belgium and Germany, which have a lower proportion of public beds. The Netherlands, however, with mainly private beds, is close to the average. There is only a weak correlation between acute beds per capita and acute admissions per capita because of large differences in average length of in-patient stay. Three countries which have reported hospital waiting lists, Ireland, Spain and the United Kingdom, all have integrated hospital systems. However, with the exception of Ireland they also have relatively low number of acute hospital beds per capita.

Inter-country comparisons of behaviour of doctors suggest other important differences, in practice, between those countries which pay physicians by fee for service and those which pay by capitation. For example, an Anglo/French comparison (Porter and Porter, 1980) suggests that French general practitioners give longer consultations, arrange more return visits, make more home visits, order more tests, prescribe more drugs and work longer hours (mainly waiting for their patients) than their British counterparts. On the other hand, they seldom work in group practices or delegate work and keep poorer records. The picture for specialists is somewhat similar. French patients seldom wait for appointments with GPs or specialists or for admission to hospital. British patients see their general practitioners fairly promptly (albeit mainly at a time of the doctors' choosing) but are frequently kept waiting many weeks both for public hospital, out-patient consultations and for public in-patient treatment. The (British) authors concluded that, "The British patient under the NHS receives skilled, delayed and often impersonal treatment. The French patient receives skilled, prompt and personal treatment".

EQUITY IN FINANCING AND DELIVERY

In Chapter 1 we put forward two equity objectives of health care policy: payment for health services in accordance with ability to pay; and treatment according to need, at least in the public sector. Of course, precise notions of equity will differ between individuals and countries. A recent study funded by the European Community on *Equity in the Finance and Delivery of Health Care* (Wagstaff *et al.,* forthcoming) measured the performance of ten health care systems against these objectives. Five of the seven countries in this report were included in the European Community study: France, Ireland, the Netherlands, Spain and the United Kingdom.

So far as the equity of the financing health care is concerned, several preliminary findings emerge: financing is mildly progressive in Ireland and in the United Kingdom; virtually proportional to income in France; and mildly regressive in Spain and in the Netherlands. An association probably exists between regressivity and the proportion of health expenditure financed privately. It has been suggested that the Dekker reforms will reduce the

Table 10.2. **Physician numbers, physician activity rates and hospital activity rates**

	Practicing physicians per 1 000 population	Consultations with GPs and specialists per head	Consultations time with GPs (minutes)	Medicines prescribed outside hospital per person	Acute hospital beds per 1 000 population	Acute hospital admissions per 100 population	Acute hospital average length of stay
	1989	Various years	Various years	1982	1989	1989	1986
Belgium	3.2	7.4	–	9.9	5.5	17.0	10.0
France	2.5	7.8[1]	14[1]	10.0[4]	5.6	20.6	7.2
Germany	2.8	10.8[1]	9[1]	11.2[4]	7.6	18.7	12.4
Ireland	1.5	6.5[2]	–	9.5	4.7	16.4	7.0
Netherlands	2.4	5.4[1]	5[1]	3.7[5]	4.8	10.4	11.5
Spain	3.5	4.2	3[3]	9.6[4]	3.5	9.0	9.7
United Kingdom	1.4	5.2[1]	8[1]	6.5	3.2	12.9[6]	7.8

1. *Source:* Sandier, 1989.
2. Public patients of GPs only, 1987. Ireland paid GPs by fee for service for such patients up to March 1989.
3. *Source:* Miguel and Guillen, 1989. Figure for 1982.
4. *Source:* O'Brien, B., 1984.
5. *Source:* IMS Netherland B.V., 1989. Figure for 1983.
6. Figures are for England and Wales and exclude the small independent sector.
Source: OECD Health Systems: *Facts and Trends*, 1993, Paris, unless otherwise stated.

Table 10.3. **Life expectancy and perinatal mortality**

| | Life expectancy at birth, 1989 | | Perinatal mortality (percentage of live and still births) | | Percentage change in perinatal mortality |
	F	M	1980	1989	1980-1989
Belgium	79.1	72.4	1.42	1.02*	−28*
France	80.6	72.5	1.29	0.89	32
Germany	79.0	72.6	1.16	0.64	45
Ireland	77.0	71.0	1.48	0.99	33
Netherlands	79.9	73.7	1.11	0.96	14
Spain	80.1**	74.5**	1.44	1.00*	−31*
United Kingdom	78.64	72.8	1.34	0.90	33

* 1987 or 1980-1987.
** 1990.
Source: OECD Health Systems: Facts and Trends, 1993, Paris.

regressivity of the payment system in the Netherlands (van Doorslaer *et al.,* forthcoming). Equity in the delivery of health care is also being examined by the European Community but the early results were too tentative to report here. The most recent evidence from the United Kingdom suggests that, in that country, the delivery of health care is broadly equitable (O'Donnell *et al.,* 1991).

HEALTH STATUS AND HEALTH OUTCOME

It is difficult to say whether variations in the levels and composition of health services affect the health of the population. Table 10.3 provides data on life expectancy and on changes in perinatal mortality for the seven countries. Variations in life expectancy can probably tell us little about the effectiveness of health services, because life expectancy is influenced by many variables apart from medical care. Spain, with the lowest health expenditure per capita of the seven countries, has average life expectancy either equal to or higher than the highest among the other countries. By contrast, variations in perinatal mortality are likely to tell us something about the effectiveness of maternity services. Perinatal mortality is the main component of "avoidable mortality" (mortality from conditions amenable to successful medical intervention – see Charlton and Velez, 1986). A sharp drop in perinatal mortality occurred between 1980 and 1987 (or 1986) in all seven countries, probably as a result of the application of new techniques for rescuing low-weight babies. Germany have led the way in this respect.

Average life expectancy can conceal differences in the dispersion of age at death, or health inequality. Legrand (1987) has pointed out that, after age standardization, less inequality in age of death occurs in the United Kingdom and Ireland than in Belgium, the Netherlands and Germany and that, in turn, these five countries, rank below Spain. France occupies either a middling rank or a high rank in terms of inequality, depending on the precise measure chosen. However, it is not clear what role, if any, health services play in these differences.

SATISFACTION WITH HEALTH CARE SYSTEMS

An important, if subjective, test of the performance of health care systems is the extent to which they satisfy consumers and taxpayers. Few international surveys of satisfaction with health care systems have been carried out. However, one recent survey of ten nations has been published by Blendon *et al.* (1990). Four of the countries in this study are included in the Blendon survey: France, the Netherlands, Germany and the United Kingdom (Spain has subsequently been added).

One measure of satisfaction which can be derived from this survey is the percentage of respondents who agreed with the statement: "On the whole, the health care system works pretty well, and only minor changes are necessary to make it work better". The results suggest relatively high levels of satisfaction (56-41% satisfied) in countries such as Canada, the Netherlands, Germany and France. These all combine moderate or high levels of per capita health expenditure with universal or near universal health insurance coverage, high levels of patient choice, and reliance, in the main, on the public contract or public reimbursement models in which "money follows the patient''. Relatively low levels of satisfaction (27-12% satisfied) are found in countries such as the United Kingdom and Italy, both of which combine low levels of per capita health expenditure with universal coverage and reliance on the public integrated model in which money does not "follow the patient''. It is not clear whether low levels of expenditure on health care or the integrated health care model are responsible for the low levels of satisfaction in the United Kingdom and Italy. To judge by the findings from Sweden (32% satisfied), a much higher level of health expenditure does little to improve the popularity of the integrated model. Unfortunately, the survey does not contain a clear example of a country which combines low levels of health expenditure with the reimbursement or contract models. The lowest level of satisfaction (only 10% satisfied) is reserved for the country with the highest level of per capita health expenditure; the United States, the only country in the survey with significant gaps in health insurance coverage.

References

Blendon, R.J., Leitman, R., Morrison, I. and Donelan, K. (1990), "Satisfaction with health systems in ten nations'', *Health Affairs,* Summer.

Charlton, J.R.H. and Velez, R. (1986), "Some International Comparisons of Mortality Amenable to Medical Intervention'', *British Medical Journal,* Vol. 292, 1 February.

Culyer, A.J. (1989), "Cost-Containment in Europe'', *Health Care Financing Review,* Annual Supplement.

Gerdtham, U.G., Sogaard, J., Jönsson, B. and Andersson, F. (1990), "A Pooled Cross-Sectional Analysis of the Health Care Expenditures of the OECD Countries'', paper prepared for the Second World Congress on Health Economics, Zurich, September.

IMS Nederland B.V., (1989), *Farmaceutische Almanak.*

Legrand, J. (1987), "Inequalities in Health: Some International Comparisons'', *European Economic Review,* Vol. 31, pp. 182-191.

Miguel, J.M. de and Guillen M.F. (1989), "The Health System in Spain'', in Field M.G. (Ed.), *Success and Crisis in National Health Systems: A Comparative Approach,* Routledge, New York.

O' Brien, B., (1984), *Patterns of European Diagnoses and Prescribing,* Office of Health Economics, London, January.

O'Donnell, O., Propper, C. and Upward, R. (1991), *An Empirical Study of Equity in the Financing and Delivery of Health Care in Britain,* Centre for Health Economics, University of York, Discussion Paper No. 85.

OECD (1987), *Financing and Delivering Health Care,* OECD, Paris.

Porter, A.M.W. and Porter J.M.T. (1980), "Anglo-French contrasts in medical practice'', *British Medical Journal,* 26 April.

Sandier, S. (1989), "Health Services Utilisation and Physician Income Trends'', *Health Care Financing Review,* Annual Supplement.

Schieber, G.J. and Poullier, J.-P. (1989), "International Health Care Expenditure Trends: 1987'', *Health Affairs,* Fall.

Wagstaff, A., van Doorslaer, E. and Rutten, F. (forthcoming), *Equity in the Finance and Delivery of Health Care,* European Community, Bruxelles.

Chapter 11

COMPARISON AND APPRAISAL OF THE REFORMS

INTRODUCTION

The purpose of this chapter is to compare and appraise the reforms which we described in Chapters 3 to 9. Our aim is to focus on the extent to which the reforms enabled governments to tackle the failures of their systems and brought them closer to meeting their policy objectives for health care. With this in mind, the discussion is organised according to a condensed version of the six main health policy objectives set out in Chapter 1:

- Adequacy, equity and income protection;
- Macro-economic efficiency;
- Micro-economic efficiency, freedom of choice for consumers, and appropriate autonomy for providers.

The discussion makes use of the seven sub-systems of public finance and delivery of health care set out in Chapter 1. The three dominant sub-systems, all of which involve compulsory, third-party finance are:

- The public reimbursement model which, in its pure form has: sickness funds, financed by compulsory, income-related contributions; which reimburse patients for out-of-pocket, fee-for-service payments to independent providers; typically with cost-sharing; but with no connection between sickness funds and providers;
- The public contract model, which in its commonest form has: sickness funds, financed by compulsory, income-related contributions; which contract directly with independent providers for services supplied free of charge to patients; and
- The public integrated model, which in its commonest form has: a public central fund, financed by general taxes; which pays doctors by salaries and public hospitals by global budgets for services supplied free of charge to patients.

Most of the seven countries rely on one, two or even three of these sub-systems, often with modifications to the pure or common form outlined above, such as the substitution of general taxation, wholly or partly, for income-related contributions, or vice versa.

Chart 11.1 summarises the main reforms discussed in Chapters 3 to 9, grouped according to the policy objectives set out above.

ADEQUACY, EQUITY AND INCOME PROTECTION

The main conclusion here is that public finance continues to be the preferred way of funding the bulk of health care in all seven countries. In most of the countries, the great majority of people were already covered by compulsory health insurance. The main exceptions were the Netherlands with about 40% voluntarily insured for acute risks, Germany with about 23% voluntarily insured (more than half of whom had joined statutory sickness funds) and Spain and Ireland with about 15% voluntarily insured for some or all acute risks.

Policy-makers heard, but did not act upon, calls made during the decade for individuals – or more individuals – to be given the freedom to opt out of compulsory systems. Rather, two of the countries, Spain and the Netherlands, extended, and announced an intention to extend, respectively, compulsory, comprehensive coverage to their entire populations. The groups which were made newly eligible, and were obliged to contribute, comprised the higher income groups and the self-employed. The reasons for including these were not so much that they lacked access to insurance coverage (most were considered good risks and were adequately served by private insurers), but that the private insurance premiums they paid were lower for given cover than the contributions paid by individuals on lesser incomes in the public system. The burden of paying for the most disadvantaged groups through social security contributions was consequently falling disproportionately on mid-

Chart 11.1 Summary of recent reforms to the health care systems of seven OECD countries

ADEQUACY, EQUITY AND INCOME PROTECTION

Extensions to compulsory insurance systems
Spain, 1984, 1986 and 1989; Netherlands, early 1990s; Ireland, 1991.

MACRO-ECONOMIC EFFICIENCY

1. Extra billing for physicians; 2. minor increases in cost-sharing
1. France, 1980; 2. most countries, various dates.

Global budgeting for physicians
Germany, 1977; Belgium, 1991.

Capitation payments for physicians
Ireland, 1989.

Global budgets for hospitals
Netherlands, 1983; Belgium, 1984; France, 1984 and 1985; Germany, 1986.

MICRO-ECONOMIC EFFICIENCY, CHOICE AND AUTONOMY

Switch from integrated model to social insurance contract model
Former Eastern Germany, 1991.

Managed competition between physicians
Germany, 1977; United Kingdom, 1990.

Managed competition between pharmaceutical products
Germany, 1989; Netherlands, 1991.

Managed competition between hospitals
Germany, 1989; United Kingdom, 1992; Netherlands, anticipated early 1990s.

Managed competition between insurers or "fundholders"
United Kingdom, 1991; Netherlands, anticipated early 1990s.

dle-income groups. The finances of the compulsory systems were also improved by including all individuals with high incomes in the schemes. Both equity and efficiency arguments may be put forward in favour of universal eligibility for basic health care, treatment according to need and contributions according to ability to pay. A widespread altruism in the case of health care is unlikely to be served satisfactorily by private charity. Moreover, to maximise the improvement in the health of the population through health services, basic medical care has to be allocated according to need (Culyer, 1989).

One implication was that voluntary insurance became increasingly supplementary in those countries which expanded their public systems. However, none adopted the Canadian policy of outlawing voluntary insurance which offered benefits already covered by the public scheme. Access to voluntary insurance was seen as an important freedom, even when, as in the French case, it was used to cover the "*ticket modérateur*", thereby removing the intended cost-consciousness at the time at which patients used services.

Concerns persisted in most countries about remaining inequities in health and in access to health care (for the United Kingdom, see Townsend and Davidson, 1982). The evidence for the former was clearer than that for the latter. The United Kingdom had instituted measures at the end of the 1970s to bring about greater geographical equity in hospital expenditure. Spain followed with similar measures in the 1980s.

MACRO-ECONOMIC EFFICIENCY AND COST-CONTAINMENT

Most OECD countries experienced unacceptably high rates of growth of medical care expenditures in the 1970s. That is to say, their governments, which were responsible for the bulk of health care expenditure, came round to the view that the opportunity costs of further increases in the taxes necessary to finance health expenditure were too high. Moreover, more than a suspicion existed in many countries that demand had been induced by suppliers. Governments took the view that reduced rates of growth of expenditure would still be capable of accommodating the most important demand pressures arising from demographic change and new medical technologies. In addition, it was also felt that health care systems could be made more efficient.

The main finding of this study is that the governments of the seven countries enjoyed much greater success in their attempts at cost-containment during the 1980s. All kept the growth rates of their health expenditure shares of GDP well below those of the previous decade. The countries which relied mainly on public contract models (systems in which public third-party funders contract directly with the providers), Germany and the Netherlands, were almost as successful as the countries which relied mainly on public integrated models (systems in which third-party funders and providers are vertically integrated in the public sector). Both were more successful than the countries which still relied partly on models which involved public reimbursement of patients. This was probably the result of the more widespread adoption of global budgets by the systems with contract models.

However, in all cases, costs were contained in the face of uncertainty about the optimum level of health expenditure and about the capacity of systems to improve their productivity. Moreover, they were contained in the face of opposition from providers and consumers. The pressures for higher health expenditure did not go away. It could be argued that some of the governments drove health spending below the optimum level, but no reliable yardstick exists by which such a shortfall could be measured and, putting aside electorates, no higher authority exists on the opportunity costs of tax-funded health expenditure than the governments themselves.

COST-SHARING IN THE PUBLICLY FINANCED SECTOR

To some extent, attempts to contain costs were made from the demand side by requiring cost-sharing in the publicly financed sector. Several of the seven countries introduced, or increased, modest compulsory co-payments and co-insurance (but not deductibles) for ambulatory and hospital services provided under the public scheme. Two countries introduced schemes which allowed negotiable cost-sharing (or extra billing). However, policy-makers generally resisted calls made at the beginning of the decade to shift a substantial part of the burden of paying for services onto patients.

This caution seemed well placed. Whereas evidence is plentiful that cost-sharing at the time at which care is utilised will reduce the level of demand for medical care – especially where the patient's income is low and where the patient has some discretion over the use of the service (van de Ven, 1983) – , it is doubtful whether reliance on anything other than modest charges (with exemptions for those with low incomes and the chronic sick) will be either equitable or efficient. It may be more efficient to encourage the doctor – who is usually the main decision-maker – to supply cost-effective care. Apart from this, consumers will often take out supplementary insurance to cover charges if not prevented from doing so.

France and Germany both introduced negotiable cost-sharing for specific services under their public schemes (at the time at which care was utilised). At the beginning of the decade, France permitted certain doctors to elect for extra billing, by allowing them to join a "sector 2" within the convention which governs medical fees. The assumption seemed to be that any extra billing would be self-limiting, because patients would prefer to consult doctors who abided by the negotiated fees. However, the result was that, by 1989, 26% of doctors had elected for extra billing, and in large cities it had become difficult to find specialists who abided by the negotiated fees. This represented a threat to access for lower income groups. In 1990, the government felt obliged to limit future elections for extra billing, provoking strikes among junior hospital doctors, many of whom aspired to join sector 2. This provides an illustration of the dangers of allowing unlimited, negotiable cost-sharing under health insurance when the supply curve is inelastic. Enthoven (1988) has pointed out that in such a situation the price tends to rise to the sum of the insurance payment and the full willingness of the patient to pay, leaving the patient, in effect, uninsured.

By contrast, Germany seems more likely to enjoy success with its recent scheme for basing sickness fund payments for certain classes of drugs (perfect substitutes for each other) on a fixed, competitive price, leaving the patient to make a contribution only if a higher priced drug in the group is chosen. Here, supply at the fixed price is likely to be perfectly elastic, with no threat to the availability of drugs for the less well-off.

Another form of restraint on the demand side is to require negotiable, extra contributions towards basic health insurance on top of compulsory insurance contributions. In many circumstances, participation by consumers in costs is preferable to cost-sharing at the time at which services are utilised, because it is negotiated and paid for when the consumer is well, rather than when he or she is sick. Negotiable extra contributions are rare in compulsory systems (putting aside supplementary insurance) because of the absence of competition. They are, however, a significant feature of the Dutch proposals for choice of insurer under their new compulsory scheme.

It is envisaged that a share of the total average premium (15% in the initial proposal) will take the form of a voluntary and transferable payment by the insured member to the insurer, which will be: specific to each insurer; flat-rate across all members; and subject to competition. The aim is that competition among insurers will exert downward pressure on the flat-rate premium which will, in turn, encourage a search for cost savings in the contracts with providers. However, it may be necessary to guard against the possibility that some insurers might make exclusive arrangements with providers in inelastic supply – for example, leading medical specialists – with a view to marketing luxury policies at premium prices. More generally, the behaviour of competitive voluntary health insurance markets does not inspire confidence in their ability to contain costs. For example, average premiums in the unregulated health insurance market in the United Kingdom rose by about 90 % in real terms between 1980 and 1988.

COST-CONTAINMENT ON THE SUPPLY SIDE

Control of health expenditure in the seven countries was achieved mainly not by increasing cost-consciousness among consumers, but by strengthening the hand of third-party payers or, in the absence of this, by imposing direct central controls on payments to providers and on the capacity of the system. There was further retreat from the pure reimbursement model, where this survived, in favour of the contract model. Within the contract model, some countries encouraged their sickness funds to act less like passive funders towards sickness funds as active purchasers, constrained by global budgets. Where command and control regulations held sway, the main instruments wielded included: fee and price controls; capacity controls (on beds and major equipment); and controls on wages and salaries in the public sector. In the integrated model, global budgets and restraint on wages and salaries were the main instruments used.

In ambulatory care, the Netherlands, Spain and the United Kingdom already had capitation payments for the public patients of general practitioners at the beginning of the period. Ireland moved from fee for service to capitation for the public patients of general practitioners during the period, and Spain moved from capitation to salary for primary care doctors. Germany adopted global budgets for aggregate payments to physicians after 1977. Belgium extended global budgets (retaining fee for service) to those parts of its system which lacked them, in 1991. Only France is still without a means of capping payments to physicians outside hospitals. Prior to the imposition of global budgets, although countries took vigorous action to contain fees, the volume of medical interventions continued to rise.

Pharmaceutical expenditure was one of the most buoyant programmes in the 1980s in all seven countries. This was the result of new developments in drugs and the absence of effective caps on expenditure or volume. Most of the countries took price control measures, and most introduced limited lists which exclude certain drugs from reimbursement. Attempts to persuade doctors to prescribe more economically, such as the Bavarian experiment, were unsuccessful, apparently because the incentives did not reward individual doctors. In 1989, Germany introduced reference pricing for drugs with strong substitutes, followed by the Netherlands in 1991; the United Kingdom announced an intention to introduce indicative prescribing budgets for general practitioners.

The most important reforms were introduced to hospital programmes. At the beginning of the period, only Ireland, Spain and the United Kingdom had global budgets for hospitals (either in aggregate or individually) but during the decade they were joined by the remaining four countries. Private hospitals were excluded in France, and budgets applied to part only of hospital expenditure in Belgium. Global budgets may be expected to work more effectively than either price or volume controls on their own, because they cannot be avoided by raising volume when price is fixed or by raising prices when volume is fixed. Local managers can be left to exercise their discretion as to how economies are made. Moreover, global budgets seem to be successful. A sustained improvement in cost control, measured by stabilization in real hospital expenditure, was achieved in the four countries for several years after global budgets were introduced. This compares with diagnosis-related group reimbursement for hospitals in the United States, which caused only a brief slowing down in the rate of growth of hospital expenditure (Pauly, 1988). Econometric analysis of per capita health expenditure across all OECD countries suggests that hospital global budgets reduce total national health expenditure by about 13%, other things being equal (Gerdtham *et al.,* 1990).

In long-term care, the United Kingdom had developed what amounted to a open-ended reimbursement programme for residential and nursing home care for the elderly, funded out of social security. In one decade, expenditure had risen over tenfold in real terms, far more rapidly than spending on domiciliary care which, ostensibly, had priority in terms of government policy. At the end of the period, the government announced an intention to: fix a budget for this programme; to put it under local authority control; to encourage authorities to set up an assessment programme for those needing long-term support to determine whether their needs would best be met by domiciliary or institutional care; to encourage the purchase of care from both the private and public sectors; and to foster consumer choice.

Global budgets and other methods for capping expenditure may be necessary conditions for sustained control of spending, but they are not sufficient. Also necessary is a determined national policy on the setting of budgets and other payments to providers. It has been said that single source financing, of the kind found in public systems financed out of general taxation, is a necessary condition for control of health expenditure. However, Germany and the Netherlands demonstrated during the 1980s that a determined government can secure cost control, even in a system with a multitude of payers, including private payers. This was done by direct central intervention in the Netherlands and by highly decentralised negotiations between sickness funds and providers under the umbrella of a "Concerted Action" programme in Germany. The econometric study cited previously (Gerdtham *et al.,* 1990) suggests that the public share of finance is itself associated with reducing costs: an increase of 1% in the public share of total health expenditure decreases per capita health expenditure by 0.23%. It seems that compulsory finance is conducive to cost control as well as equity. Nevertheless, the Dutch example shows that a determined government can control even voluntary health expenditure.

COST-CONTAINMENT IN THE VOLUNTARILY FINANCED SECTOR

There were noticeable differences in the development of regulation of voluntary insurers between those countries where part of the population relied on voluntary health insurance for all or part of basic medical care, and those where voluntary insurance was entirely supplementary. Thus, private insurers in the Netherlands were increasingly heavily regulated with controls on premiums and the introduction of some mandatory open enrolment. In Ireland, voluntary insurance is provided under a statutory monopoly which has exercised increasing discipline over providers. In contrast, competing private insurers remained virtually unregulated in the United Kingdom where public coverage was universal. Between 1980 and 1988, average premiums rose by about 45% in real terms in Ireland and by about 90 % in the United Kingdom – at a time when the real, average cost of acute hospital care per capita in the national health service hardly changed at all. Governments presumably consider *laisser faire* to be entirely appropriate when health insurance plays only a supplementary role. Meanwhile, the signs are that the private market will eventually encourage the same switch away from the pure reimbursement model that has occurred in public systems. In the United Kingdom, as in the United States, competition appears to be encouraging indemnity insurers to control providers through measures such as preferred provider arrangements, managed care and utilisation reviews.

MICRO-ECONOMIC EFFICIENCY, CONSUMER CHOICE AND PROVIDER AUTONOMY

One major conclusion of this study is that micro-economic inefficiency emerged increasingly as the outstanding problem in the publicly financed health sectors of the seven countries, not least because of its link with failure of cost-containment. Ideas about improving micro-economic efficiency differed across countries. Broadly, divergence in policies emerged between those countries which continued to pin their faith on command-and-control methods, including improvements to the integrated model where relevant, and those which sought to strengthen or to introduce pro-market or quasi-market regulations and incentives. All seven could agree on the need for more quality assurance and for better information on health outcome and costs.

Each of the seven health care systems had rather different concerns about efficiency. The evidence which exists does not suggest that the systems differ in their medical effectiveness. We have seen, for example, that perinatal mortality fell sharply at about the same rate in all seven countries during the 1980s. Perinatal mobidity is a condition where the indications are usually clear. However, evidence is growing about inexplicable variations between and within countries in care for conditions where the indications are less clear. It is hard to believe that these different levels of care are all equally effective.

Where reliance has been placed on the reimbursement or contract models, and "money follows the patient", some concern is usually expressed about unnecessary care and supplier-induced demand. There is also concern about excessive regulation – often the by-product of cost-containment measures where third parties have been confined to the role of passive payment offices. Despite these concerns, countries with such arrangements seem to be relatively successful at satisfying their consumers.

Those countries with have public integrated systems, in which money does not "follow the patient", tend to become concerned about under-service and inflexible and ineffective management systems. They tend, also, to have patients who are less satisfied. It seems that (non-competitive) capitation payments and salary payments for general practitioners and specialists are sometimes associated with brisk, inconvenient and infrequent consultations. There also seems to be a link between long-established global budgets for hospitals, lacking an element of work-related payment, and waiting lists and impersonal care.

Although Belgium, France, Germany and the Netherlands have now introduced global budgets for hospitals, to some extent, money still "follows the patient" in these countries. Belgium and the Netherlands still have fee-for-service payment for hospital doctors. France has many private hospitals which offer elective surgery to public patients, where both the doctor and the hospital are paid by fee for service. And Germany has retained some links between global budgets and volume.

SOLUTIONS ADOPTED

The most sudden and dramatic reform was the wholesale conversion, during 1991, of the state health care system in Eastern Germany (before reunification) to a social insurance contract system which corresponded to that which had existed in the whole of Germany prior to the end of World War Two. This represented a decisive choice in favour of the contract model throughout a reunited Germany.

Meanwhile, more gradual but equally important reforms were under way in the Netherlands and in the United Kingdom. Those in the United Kingdom could also be described as a movement away from the public integrated model towards a version of the public contract model. The reforms in the Netherlands involved strengthening the contract model and moving beyond it, by introducing competition between insurers within a universal social insurance system. Both countries aimed at placing more reliance on self-regulating, managed market arrangements in their health care systems. Germany already had some elements of these, which were strengthened during the decade.

These three examples of managed markets all occur in countries with a strong central commitment to widespread or universal public cover for health expenses, to equitable arrangements for health care delivery in the public sector, and to tight, overall control of the level of health expenditure. Indeed, it could be argued that it is precisely the firmness of their external constraints which has permitted them to adopt the freedoms of the market within their publicly funded systems. Within this central framework, they differ significantly in the type of decentralised market structures which they have developed or are in the process of developing.

German arrangements (Chart 11.2) contain a mixture of consumer-led competition among providers, with bilateral monopoly involving the setting by the sickness funds of global budgets for providers. Germany's many sickness funds are, effectively, small monopolies. Although minimum benefits are standardized across the system, contributions vary widely. There is consumer choice between first-level doctors involving transferable fees. These adjust automatically downwards if aggregate volume increases, because global budgets are negotiated at a regional level between associations of sickness funds and of physicians. The pricing of pharmaceuticals has recently been made more competitive. Some consumer choice is available as between hospitals, and hospital budgets are responsive, to some extent, to volume. However, the dominant influence is that global budgets are set in bilateral monopoly negotiations at a regional level between the associations of sickness funds and the hospitals. Elements of competition, or potential competition, have been introduced between hospitals by improved comparisons of costs and by giving the sickness funds the right to terminate contracts. However, it is not yet clear how effectively this right will be utilised. There is separation between sickness funds and providers, although about

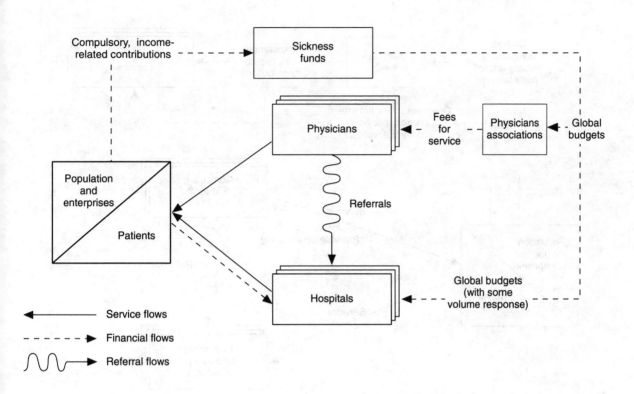

half the hospitals are in the public sector. In general, a high level of consumer choice prevails and sickness funds have the potential to play a role as sponsors of consumers.

The Netherlands (Chart 11.3) should implement, over several years, consumer-led competition among insurers and a mixture of consumer-led and insurer-led competition between providers. A central fund will convert income-related contributions collected under social insurance into risk-related premiums paid to independent insurers. This will enable consumers to choose their insurer without the resulting competition providing incentives for insurers to practise risk selection. This amounts to a sophisticated voucher scheme. With a view to fostering cost-conscious choice of insurer, the premiums will include an element of cost-sharing. Consumer choice between first-level doctors will involve (at least initially) transferable capitation fees negotiated by insurers with doctors. The hospital market seems likely to evolve in a competitive direction (mergers allowing). Already, a high level of autonomy exists among hospitals, most of which are private. It is possible that health maintenance organisation-type bodies will emerge.

The United Kingdom (Chart 11.4) plans to set up, over several years, a version of the public contract model for hospital care. This will involve separation between district health authority purchasers, funded by weighted capitation payments, and competing hospital providers, public and private. Well-managed public hospitals will be encouraged to become self-governing trusts. The United Kingdom is also planning (uniquely) to give some of its first-level doctors command over some of the funds destined for hospitals, enabling them to become active purchasers on behalf of their patients. At the same time, greater competition is to be encouraged among general practitioners. The combination of fund-holding general practitioners and competition will, in effect, mean that some consumers are being offered a partial choice of insurer under the national health service. Under these new arrangements, the government will retain direct line-management responsibility for district health authority purchasers (but GP fundholders will be independent) and will seek to regulate providers, mainly by pro-competition policies. However, the government will also retain control of capital investments in public hospitals and trusts.

What is (or will be) common to all these systems is that providers (and in the case of the Netherlands, insurers) are encouraged to satisfy consumers because there is consumer choice backed up by transferable fees,

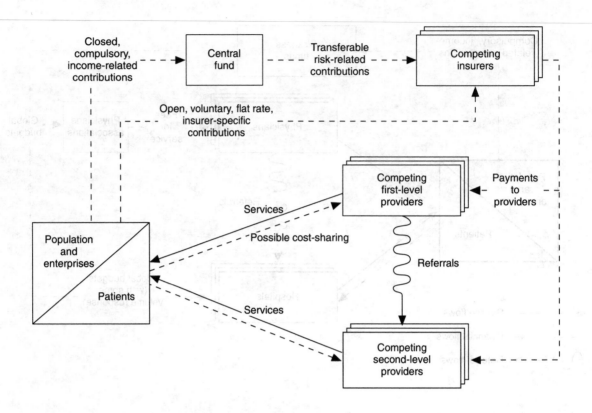

capitation payments or premiums. Money follows the patient. Local purchasers, either third-party funders or general practitioners, can act as the sponsors of consumers and negotiate over quality and cost with competing providers for the purchase of services out of limited public budgets. This will involve working out ways in which the third-party funders and the first-level doctors can co-ordinate their purchasing and referral decisions, respectively. The buyers may also assume a role which involves making distributional judgments (assessment of relative needs, especially among those with chronic illness) except in the Netherlands, where, presumably, this role will be played by the central fund.

In all three countries, the emphasis of government regulation is also switching away from command-and-control measures towards pro-competition policies. Firm macro-economic control combined with competition (or bilateral monopoly) can allow governments to stand back somewhat.

Managed markets of the kind described above offer prospects for increased consumer choice, producer autonomy and efficiency in the health systems concerned, without sacrifices in overall cost control or equity. Such arrangements will challenge the sweeping statement of Enthoven and Kronick (1989) that, "None of the countries that have adopted global budgets in the public sector have solved the problem of creating incentives for the efficient organisation and delivery of care".

Managed markets within public health care systems are, however, still relatively untried. A number of important questions still remain to be answered, for example:

– Is it possible to produce the desired improvements in efficiency in quasi markets, where both the buyers and the providers are public bodies, as is proposed in the United Kingdom? How is the government to reconcile potential disharmony between its decentralised buyers and its decentralised hospital provider/investors, for example, without becoming involved in detailed planning and appraisal of investments or of buying decisions? In these circumstances, will this form of public contract model collapse into the public integrated model?

– What are the merits of competition versus monopsony among third-party funders in the public and, indeed, considering Ireland, in the private sector?

Chart 11.4 **The reformed health care system in the United Kingdom**
(publicly financed sector)

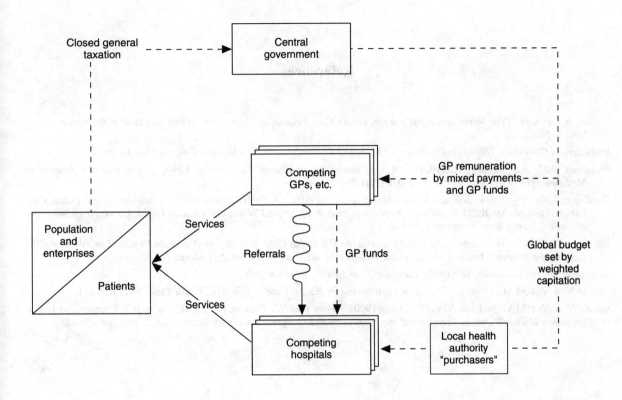

- What is the right level of competition among providers? Will the threat of competition and yardstick comparisons suffice where supply is monopolistic?
- How is it best to co-ordinate consumer choice, first-level doctor choice and third-party negotiations in the market for hospital services?
- To what extent will transaction costs erode the savings which result from adopting market incentives?
- What is the ability of the central fund to devise risk-adjusted premiums and regulations which will sufficiently discourage risk selection (or ''cream skimming'') by insurers (van de Ven, 1990). An identical dilemma is faced by Medicare in the United States in devising weighted capitation payments to allow beneficiaries to enrol in health maintenance organisations without facing risk selection.
- What is the ability of the system to secure adequate measurement of the outcome and quality of care to ensure that competition does not take place at the expense of outcome and quality?
- Will the market produce the right level of information, or will government have to step in to require disclosure and transparency, as well as to fill gaps?

As it will be some years before we will see the full effects of the reforms in the Netherlands and in the United Kingdom, we are unlikely to have authoritative answers to these questions in the near future.

References

Culyer, A.J. (1989), "The Normative Economics of Health Care Finance and Provision", *Oxford Review of Economic Policy*, Vol. 5, No. 1.

Enthoven, A.C. (1988), *Theory and Practice of Managed Competition in Health Care Finance*, Amsterdam.

Enthoven, A.C. and Kronick, R. (1989), "A Consumer Choice Health Plan for the 1990s", *New England Journal of Medicine*, Vol. 320, Nos. 1 (Part 1) and 2 (Part 2).

Gerdtham, U-G., Sogaard, J., Jonsson, B. and Andersson, F. (1990), "A Pooled Cross-Sectional Analysis of the Health Care Expenditures of the OECD Countries", paper presented at the Second World Congress on Health Economics, University of Zurich, Switzerland, September 10-14.

Pauly, M.V. (1988), "Efficiency, Equity and Costs in the US health Care System", in *American Health Care, What are the Lessons for Britain?*, Institute of Economic Affairs, Health Unit, paper No. 5, London.

Townsend, P. and Davidson, N. (1982), *Inequalities in Health*, Penguin.

van de Ven, W.P.M.M., (1983), "Effects of cost-sharing in Health Care", *Effective Health Care*, Vol. 1, No. 1.

van de Ven, W.P.M.M. and van Vliet, R.C.J.A. (1990), "How Can We Prevent Cream Skimming in a Competitive Health Insurance Market?", paper presented at the Second World Congress on Health Economics, September, Zurich.

Chapter 12

CONCLUSIONS

A number of clear conclusions emerge from this study of the reform of health care systems in seven OECD countries: some about the problems which led to the reforms being introduced; some about the content of the reforms themselves; some about the results of the reforms; and some about continuing uncertainty. However, we must be cautious about offering firm policy recommendations on the basis of this study for several reasons:

- Although countries share similar objectives for their health care systems, the weights which they attach to these objectives may differ;
- Most health care systems are made up from only a few, common sub-systems, which helps us to compare experience across frontiers. However, no two countries share exactly the same mix of sub-systems and it is possible that there are different interactions between different sub-systems which will limit the possibility for making valid transfers of experience;
- Although it may be possible to offer technical experience across frontiers, this will be of little use if a country faces insurmountable political obstacles to change;
- Some of the most important reforms described, particularly those in the Netherlands and the United Kingdom, involve experimentation with new mechanisms whose full effects will not become clear until long after this report has been published.

The conclusions are, once again, constructed around the condensed list of the policy objectives for health care set out in Chapter 11, and around the dominant sub-systems for financing and delivering health care set out in Chapter 1.

ADEQUACY, EQUITY AND INCOME PROTECTION

Public finance remained the preferred way of funding access to basic health care for the great majority of people in all seven countries, despite calls in some quarters for more reliance on voluntary coverage. No country reduced coverage by the public sector and two countries, Spain and the Netherlands, respectively made, and announced an intention to make, compulsory coverage universal. Voluntary health insurance had become, or was to become, supplementary in most of the seven countries. Cost-sharing in the public system also remained modest or very modest in all of the countries.

A number of plausible explanations may be advanced for the attachment of these European countries to solidarity in health care, including: widespread and strong feelings of altruism among their populations towards the sick; and the perception that treatment according to need rather than according to ability to pay is likely to maximise the sum of improvements to health that can be brought about by any given share of GDP which is devoted to health expenditure.

That is not to say that public systems have always succeeded in achieving the intended level of equity in payment for or access to health care within the public system. For example, differentials in contributions for similar benefits persist among sickness funds in Germany, and some continuing differentials in access to services for given needs have been recorded in several countries. However, these differentials are a great deal less than they would have been under voluntary systems. More important are the intractable and persistent differentials in health status which occur across socio-economic groups in all of the countries. It is beyond the power of health care systems on their own to remove these differentials.

MACRO-ECONOMIC EFFICIENCY

There are two important implications for universal or near universal public financing of medical care. First, because consumers are no longer conscious of costs, they have incentives to demand more than the optimum level of health care, and providers, especially if payment for their services is work-related, have incentives to supply this. Second, governments become responsible for exercising restraint and for setting the level of the bulk of health expenditure. In discharging this awesome responsibility, governments face two difficulties: a coalition of consumer and producer interests which is opposed to restraint and genuine uncertainty about the correct level of health expenditure.

The governments of all the seven countries enjoyed increasing success with cost-containment in the late 1970s and 1980s. Their health expenditure shares of GDP grew more slowly, stopped growing, or in the case of Ireland, were reduced. This success was particularly marked in the two countries with sickness funds, and which relied mainly on the public contract model (Germany and the Netherlands) as well as in the three countries which relied on general tax finance and mainly integrated provision (Ireland, Spain and the United Kingdom). Success with cost-containment was slightly less in evidence in the two countries which still relied to some extent on the public reimbursement model (Belgium and France). The strong suggestion is that any cost-containment was achieved not by the modest increases in cost-sharing that took place (the cost-containment intentions of which were, anyhow, sometimes circumvented by voluntary health insurance) but by direct action on the supply side, either by strengthening the hand of the third-party payers through, for example, the introduction of global budgeting, or by direct central regulation of fees and charges. Global budgets were introduced in parts of the Belgian and French systems during the period, diminishing the extent to which they relied on demand-led, open-ended reimbursement of patients. The Netherlands relied for cost-containment both on global budgets for hospitals and on direct, central regulation of providers.

A not surprising conclusion would be that the public reimbursement model is less suited to achieving cost-containment than the public contract and integrated models. The same is observed to be the case with the voluntary versions of these models in the United States: private indemnity insurance compared with various types of health maintenance organisation. And, indeed, although Belgium and France still adhere to some of the procedures of the reimbursement model, they have increasingly had recourse to direct negotiations between sickness funds and providers (the contract model) or, in the case of public hospitals in France, to direct expenditure controls through public control and ownership (the integrated model).

MICRO-ECONOMIC EFFICIENCY, CONSUMER CHOICE AND PROVIDER AUTONOMY

The objective of micro-economic efficiency in health care includes the idea of raising static efficiency: that is, improving value for money (where the value to be maximised is some combination of the health status of the population and satisfaction with the process of medical care, to be weighted by judgments about social welfare). It also includes the idea of dynamic efficiency: that is, improvements over time in medical and organisational techniques which raise the productivity of scarce human and physical resources. It is likely that, over time, gains from technological change will outweigh those which result from improvements in static efficiency.

Agreement is less widespread about how to achieve these micro-economic objectives than about how to achieve the coverage and cost-containment objectives discussed above, for several reasons:

- we still lack adequate measures of the outcome and quality of care which hampers the measurement of efficiency;
- differences of view remain on how best to motivate health care providers, especially doctors, to act in a cost-effective fashion;
- as has been mentioned above, we still await the results of the important reforms, which are directed mainly at efficiency problems, in the Netherlands and the United Kingdom.

The previous chapter shows that some dissatisfaction remains with the micro-economic performance of the public integrated model. Although there can be, and often is, patient choice (under medical advice) when public hospitals are funded by global budgets and doctors are salaried, the exercise of choice does not lead to financial rewards for successful providers at the expense of unsuccessful providers. In other words, money does not follow the patient. Similar complaints are attached to capitation payment combined with restraints on competition. The integrated model seems to be associated with waiting lists and patients who are grateful supplicants rather than empowered consumers. And while medical innovation does not seem to be discouraged – so long as doctors enjoy clinical freedom – the integrated model does appear to discourage organisational innovation. It should be noted that steps towards abandoning this model have been taken recently; not only in the United Kingdom and in Eastern Germany, but also elsewhere in Central and Eastern Europe, in Sweden and in the former USSR.

The reforms in the United Kingdom involve: the strengthening of consumer-led competition between general practitioners; the handing over of some of the funds destined for hospital care to large GP practices; the separation of the buying of hospital care by local health authorities from the provision of care; enabling well-managed public hospitals to become self-governing; and encouraging competition for public funds from private hospitals. Subject to the development of suitable contracts, these changes will encourage the emergence of a market or quasi-market for hospital care in which money will follow patient choice (under the advice of general practitioners). This involves a move towards the public contract model in the hospital market, albeit with few independent hospitals, at least initially.

The previous chapter shows also that there is disillusionment in several countries with command and control regulation of health care. Reliance on command and control regulation arose in some countries with the integrated model and in others from cost-control measures in public reimbursement and contract systems, devoted to market principles. Public integrated systems also find it difficult to escape centralisation tendencies despite attempts to delegate managerial discretion to local public health authorities. However, German experience suggests that the public contract model is suitable for considerable self-regulation under a firm central policy of expenditure control. This is because of the countervailing power that can be established between local sickness funds and local providers. The reforms in the United Kingdom and the Netherlands offer prospects of a similar degree of self-regulation through pro-competition regulation. It should be emphasized that their governments will still need to set the expenditure framework and to regulate the policy of the public buyers, as well as the operation of the market. The aim is to allow governments to stand back, not to abdicate the field entirely.

COMBINING EFFICIENCY AND EQUITY IN PROVIDER MARKETS

One clear implication of the discussion above is that the public contract model combines more desirable features than either the public reimbursement or the public integrated models. The reimbursement model lacks adequate mechanisms for cost-containment, putting aside unacceptable levels of cost-sharing. The integrated model lacks (financial) incentives for micro-economic efficiency, given that money does not "follow the patient". Only the contract model is suited *both* to the pursuit of macro-economic efficiency *and* to the pursuit of micro-economic efficiency. In addition, the contract model seems better suited to self-regulation and appropriate provider autonomy than either of the other two models.

In view of this, it is not surprising that there are some signs of convergence on the contract model among the seven countries. Belgium has moved away from the public reimbursement model towards the public contract model. The Netherlands is expected to reduce its reliance on the voluntary reimbursement model. The United Kingdom and Eastern Germany have moved away from the integrated model towards the contract model.

Some new varieties of contract model are emerging from the reforms. In the case of first-level providers, it is normal for the third parties to play a relatively passive and enabling role, allowing competition to be led by consumers. The question remains as to whether it is better to pay primary care doctors by capitation or by fee for service, or by some mix of the two, as in the United Kingdom. In the case of hospital care, more choices are available. The third-party payer can be a public or quasi-public monopoly insurer, such as a sickness fund, or it can be the primary care gatekeeper, as with the GP "fundholders" in the United Kingdom. Where the third-party payer for hospital is not the primary care doctor, choices are available as to whether this body is a relatively passive funder following, rather than leading, the referral patterns of primary care doctors – or is a relatively active purchaser. The second role seems particularly appropriate where questions are raised about the distribution of public expenditure among major patient groups – for example, those in need of acute hospital care and those in need of long-term hospital care. There are choices as to how global budgets are combined with work-related payment systems for hospitals. There are also choices as to: whether public third parties confine their contracts to public hospitals, creating an "internal" market (Enthoven and Kronick, 1985); whether hospitals become or remain independent; or whether a mixture of hospitals is envisaged, as in the emerging system in the United Kingdom. It remains to be seen how competition will work out in practice in those systems where the public sector has an interest in both sides of the market.

A further finding which emerges from this study concerns the growing number of examples of "mixed" forms of payment of providers within public contract systems. These combine an overall expenditure cap with rewards for the productivity of individual providers. Examples include:

- capitation and competition (general practitioners in Ireland, the Netherlands and the United Kingdom);
- global budgets and fee for service (physicians in Germany);

149

– global budgets and volume-related contracts (hospitals in Germany and the United Kingdom).

Mixed methods of payment are capable of transmitting signals to providers both about benefits and about cost-constraints.

It is interesting to note that three authors who have explored the theoretical characteristics of optimal payment systems for health services in the United States, have concluded that, "Payment systems that achieve the desired balance between protecting consumers from financial risk and controlling costs are characterised by generous insurance coverage and financial incentives on providers to control costs." The best financial incentives for providers appear to be "... mixed (payment) system(s)... with some part of payment prospective and some part of payment cost based." (Ellis and McGuire, 1990). Alternatively, the payment system may be a mixture of capitation and partial reimbursement of provider costs (Selden, 1990). Also, "... supply based policies are the preferred instruments for cost control ... cost based reimbursement is never part of an optimal health care payment system" (Ellis and McGuire, 1990).

If equity objectives as well as efficiency objectives are to be well served in a partly self-regulating contract model, it is desirable to have a central fund for equalising contribution rates (if the source of finance is not general taxation) and for allocating risk-related aggregate budgets to decentralised third-party funding bodies. Budgets should be based on the population to be served by the funding bodies, weighted for factors such as age structure and relative morbidity (or mortality). It may also be desirable for the third-party funding bodies to establish purchasing budgets for different need groups among the population and to act as active "buyers" on behalf of these groups.

It is an interesting exercise to list what might be said to be the ideal features of the partly self-regulating, public contract model or public provider market. Clearly, none of the seven countries in this study yet has such a model fully in operation. Experimentation and development are still under way, particularly in the United Kingdom. However, all of the following key components seem to have been tried out or tested already in one or other of the seven countries, although not all at the same time and in the same place:

– universal public cover with supplementary voluntary insurance (Belgium, France, United Kingdom);
– government control of total public health expenditure (Germany, Netherlands, United Kingdom);
– a central fund for allocating risk-related budgets to decentralised, public, monopsony, third-party funding bodies (Belgium, United Kingdom);
– decentralised funding bodies to establish budgets for different need groups (United Kingdom);
– separation between decentralised "buyers" and providers (Germany);
– consumer-led competition between public and private providers (France);
– globally budgeted contracts between "buyers" and providers which allow money to follow the patient (Germany);
– a high level of self-regulation by third parties and providers (Germany).

The suggestion, here, is that establishing a provider market under the public contract model is not a high-risk strategy, since most or all its components have already been tested in one country or another.

COMBINING EFFICIENCY AND EQUITY IN BOTH INSURANCE AND PROVIDER MARKETS

The Dutch reforms go beyond managed provider markets by establishing, in addition, markets for health insurance (possibly excluding long-term care) with consumer-led competition. A somewhat similar mechanism is being adopted in the United Kingdom with some of the acute hospital budget being allocated to large, competing, GP practices. The three public models presented here cannot depict such arrangements adequately. Indeed, the Dutch model (Chart 11.3) must be considered to be a new, eighth model to be added to the list of seven models set out in Chapter 1. This amounts to a sophisticated voucher scheme for health insurance. Moreover, it could be said to serve a new objective: autonomy of insurer. In this way, it involves a major extension of self-regulation beyond that involved in the provider market. In principle, this will allow consumers to choose between the three *voluntary* models of health financing and delivery, set out in Chapter 1, under the umbrella of a compulsory health insurance system. The respective roles of the reimbursement, contract and integrated models will be decided in the market.

The Dutch model could be said to involve three new key components, to add to the list for the provider model, above:

– a central fund for granting risk-related insurance premiums for acute health care to individual consumers;
– negotiable sharing in premiums by individuals;

– consumer-led competition between different insurers.

The last of these has been well tried, not only in the United States, where the arrangements for individuals to choose indemnity insurance or health maintenance organisations under Medicare resemble the Dutch model, but also in the recent and more distant past in the Netherlands itself. The first two mechanisms are relatively untried, however. If risk adjustment of premiums is inadequate, insurers will have a strong incentive to "cream skim". That is to say, they will have an incentive to compete not by becoming more efficient, but by insuring the healthier individuals who represent good risks. And it is possible to conceive that the negotiable part of the premium could have the perverse and unintended effect of enabling high-income consumers to bid health care resources away from low-income consumers. A recent American judgment on models of the Dutch kind is gloomy:

"Extensive research in Medicare and private settings has found no reliable way to measure and correct for risk selection sufficiently to make the domino theory work" (Jones, 1990).

By the "domino" theory, Jones means cost-conscious choice of insurer leading to cost-conscious choice of provider. However, there are new ideas for solving the problem of "cream skimming" by a combination of: risk-adjustment; risk-sharing between the insurers and the central fund; and pro-competition rules (van de Ven, 1990). The hope is that the intensive efforts now being devoted to this problem in the Netherlands, the United States and the United Kingdom will produce the design for a health insurance market which will allow equity and efficiency to be combined.

EPILOGUE

In several respects, the seven countries seem to be converging in their health care policies and institutions. This is evident in: the continuing moves towards universal public coverage; the strengthening of control over total health expenditure by governments; the universal adoption of global budgets in hospital markets; and in the movements towards the contract model in several countries. However, there is currently divergence on the subject of regulation. Whereas, at the beginning of the 1980s, six of the seven countries relied on a highly centralised command-and-control approach to regulation, by the end of the 1980s the Netherlands and the United Kingdom had followed Germany, by moving towards a greater measure of self-regulation.

In the case of these three countries, it might be said that they are trying to create a new division of labour between government and the market in the regulation of health care systems. Governments will be responsible for: setting the level of the bulk of health expenditure; ensuring universal, or near universal coverage for health expenses; arranging equity and distributional matters; setting the rules which govern the operations of the market; and ensuring the adequacy and transparency of information. The market will be responsible for all other matters which concern the local financing and provision of care.

Managed markets represent a new attempt to fulfil the adequacy, equity and efficiency objectives of health policy set out at the beginning of this report. However, certain trade-offs cannot be escaped: between responsiveness and equity, for example; and between cost-containment and choice. All we can hope for is that, by raising the productivity of health care systems, the reformed systems will ease the pain involved in such trade-offs.

In addition, certain intractable problems remain, especially in the field of information. The Netherlands and the United Kingdom are handicapped by the lack of an adequate methodology for adjusting capitation payments or insurance premiums for risk. All seven countries lack adequate information on the marginal product of health expenditure, to inform the difficult decisions which governments must take on the level of public health expenditure. And, above all, OECD countries lack adequate ways of measuring health outcome and the quality of care, although there are some promising signs of progress.

FURTHER WORK

The results of this study suggest a need for further work. Topics which might usefully be covered by future OECD projects include:

– further monitoring of the recent major reforms which have taken place in the Netherlands and the United Kingdom;
– analysis and appraisal of health care reforms in OECD countries not included in this study;
– more detailed international comparisons of individual sub-sectors of health care systems, particularly hospitals, pharmaceuticals, long-term care and dentistry;

- comparative analysis of how judgments are made about the distribution of public funds between different need groups;
- the advantages and disadvantages of encouraging provider competition on price and quality, instead of on quality alone;
- further work on the relatively neglected topic of international comparisons of methods of financing and planning capital investment in hospitals and mechanisms for deciding on closures;
- more co-operation among OECD Member countries to tackle the information deficiencies mentioned above.

References

Blendon, R.J., Leitman, R., Morrison, I. and Donelan, K. (1990), "Satisfaction with health systems in ten nations", *Health Affairs,* Summer.

Ellis, R.P. and McGuire, T.G. (1986), "Provider behaviour under prospective reimbursement", *Journal of Health Economics,* 5.

Ellis, R.P. and McGuire, T.G. (1990), "Optimal Payment Systems for Health Services", *Journal of Health Economics,* 9, pp. 375-396.

Enthoven, A.C. (1985), *Reflections on the Management of the National Health Service,* Nuffield Provincial Hospitals Trust.

Enthoven, A.C. and Kronick, R. (1989), "A Consumer Choice Health Plan for the 1990s", *New England Journal of Medicine,* Vol. 320, No. 1 (Part 1) and 2 (Part 2).

Jones, S.B. (1990), "Multiple choice health insurance: the lessons and challenge to private insurers", *Inquiry,* 27, Summer.

Selden, T.M. (1990), "A Model of Capitation", *Journal of Health Economics,* 9, pp. 397-409.

van de Ven, W.P.M.M. (1990), "How can we prevent cream skimming in a competitive health insurance market?", paper presented at the Second World Congress on Health Economics, September, Zurich.

MAIN SALES OUTLETS OF OECD PUBLICATIONS
PRINCIPAUX POINTS DE VENTE DES PUBLICATIONS DE L'OCDE

ARGENTINA – ARGENTINE
Carlos Hirsch S.R.L.
Galería Güemes, Florida 165, 4° Piso
1333 Buenos Aires   Tel. (1) 331.1787 y 331.2391
Telefax: (1) 331.1787

AUSTRALIA – AUSTRALIE
D.A. Book (Aust.) Pty. Ltd.
648 Whitehorse Road, P.O.B 163
Mitcham, Victoria 3132   Tel. (03) 873.4411
Telefax: (03) 873.5679

AUSTRIA – AUTRICHE
Gerold & Co.
Graben 31
Wien I   Tel. (0222) 533.50.14

BELGIUM – BELGIQUE
Jean De Lannoy
Avenue du Roi 202
B-1060 Bruxelles   Tel. (02) 538.51.69/538.08.41
Telefax: (02) 538.08.41

CANADA
Renouf Publishing Company Ltd.
1294 Algoma Road
Ottawa, ON K1B 3W8   Tel. (613) 741.4333
Telefax: (613) 741.5439
Stores:
61 Sparks Street
Ottawa, ON K1P 5R1   Tel. (613) 238.8985
211 Yonge Street
Toronto, ON M5B 1M4   Tel. (416) 363.3171
Les Éditions La Liberté Inc.
3020 Chemin Sainte-Foy
Sainte-Foy, PQ G1X 3V6   Tel. (418) 658.3763
Telefax: (418) 658.3763

Federal Publications
165 University Avenue
Toronto, ON M5H 3B8   Tel. (416) 581.1552
Telefax: (416) 581.1743

CHINA – CHINE
China National Publications Import
Export Corporation (CNPIEC)
16 Gongti E. Road, Chaoyang District
P.O. Box 88 or 50
Beijing 100704 PR   Tel. (01) 506.6688
Telefax: (01) 506.3101

DENMARK – DANEMARK
Munksgaard Export and Subscription Service
35, Nørre Søgade, P.O. Box 2148
DK-1016 København K   Tel. (33) 12.85.70
Telefax: (33) 12.93.87

FINLAND – FINLANDE
Akateeminen Kirjakauppa
Keskuskatu 1, P.O. Box 128
00100 Helsinki   Tel. (358 0) 12141
Telefax: (358 0) 121.4441

FRANCE
OECD/OCDE
Mail Orders/Commandes par correspondance:
2, rue André-Pascal
75775 Paris Cedex 16   Tel. (33-1) 45.24.82.00
Telefax: (33-1) 45.24.85.00   or (33-1) 45.24.81.76
Telex: 640048 OCDE

OECD Bookshop/Librairie de l'OCDE :
33, rue Octave-Feuillet
75016 Paris   Tel. (33-1) 45.24.81.67
(33-1) 45.24.81.81

Documentation Française
29, quai Voltaire
75007 Paris   Tel. 40.15.70.00
Gibert Jeune (Droit-Économie)
6, place Saint-Michel
75006 Paris   Tel. 43.25.91.19

Librairie du Commerce International
10, avenue d'Iéna
75016 Paris   Tel. 40.73.34.60
Librairie Dunod
Université Paris-Dauphine
Place du Maréchal de Lattre de Tassigny
75016 Paris   Tel. 47.27.18.56
Librairie Lavoisier
11, rue Lavoisier
75008 Paris   Tel. 42.65.39.95
Librairie L.G.D.J. - Montchrestien
20, rue Soufflot
75005 Paris   Tel. 46.33.89.85
Librairie des Sciences Politiques
30, rue Saint-Guillaume
75007 Paris   Tel. 45.48.36.02
P.U.F.
49, boulevard Saint-Michel
75005 Paris   Tel. 43.25.83.40
Librairie de l'Université
12a, rue Nazareth
13100 Aix-en-Provence   Tel. (16) 42.26.18.08
Documentation Française
165, rue Garibaldi
69003 Lyon   Tel. (16) 78.63.32.23
Librairie Decitre
29, place Bellecour
69002 Lyon   Tel. (16) 72.40.54.54

GERMANY – ALLEMAGNE
OECD Publications and Information Centre
Schedestrasse 7
D-W 5300 Bonn 1   Tel. (0228) 21.60.45
Telefax: (0228) 26.11.04

GREECE – GRÈCE
Librairie Kauffmann
Mavrokordatou 9
106 78 Athens   Tel. 322.21.60
Telefax: 363.39.67

HONG-KONG
Swindon Book Co. Ltd.
13–15 Lock Road
Kowloon, Hong Kong   Tel. 366.80.31
Telefax: 739.49.75

ICELAND – ISLANDE
Mál Mog Menning
Laugavegi 18, Pósthólf 392
121 Reykjavik   Tel. 162.35.23

INDIA – INDE
Oxford Book and Stationery Co.
Scindia House
New Delhi 110001   Tel.(11) 331.5896/5308
Telefax: (11) 332.5993
17 Park Street
Calcutta 700016   Tel. 240832

INDONESIA – INDONÉSIE
Pdii-Lipi
P.O. Box 269/JKSMG/88
Jakarta 12790   Tel. 583467
Telex: 62 875

IRELAND – IRLANDE
TDC Publishers – Library Suppliers
12 North Frederick Street
Dublin 1   Tel. 74.48.35/74.96.77
Telefax: 74.84.16

ISRAEL
Electronic Publications only
Publications électroniques seulement
Sophist Systems Ltd.
71 Allenby Street
Tel-Aviv 65134   Tel. 3-29.00.21
Telefax: 3-29.92.39

ITALY – ITALIE
Libreria Commissionaria Sansoni
Via Duca di Calabria 1/1
50125 Firenze   Tel. (055) 64.54.15
Telefax: (055) 64.12.57
Via Bartolini 29
20155 Milano   Tel. (02) 36.50.83
Editrice e Libreria Herder
Piazza Montecitorio 120
00186 Roma   Tel. 679.46.28
Telefax: 678.47.51
Libreria Hoepli
Via Hoepli 5
20121 Milano   Tel. (02) 86.54.46
Telefax: (02) 805.28.86
Libreria Scientifica
Dott. Lucio de Biasio 'Aeiou'
Via Coronelli, 6
20146 Milano   Tel. (02) 48.95.45.52
Telefax: (02) 48.95.45.48

JAPAN – JAPON
OECD Publications and Information Centre
Landic Akasaka Building
2-3-4 Akasaka, Minato-ku
Tokyo 107   Tel. (81.3) 3586.2016
Telefax: (81.3) 3584.7929

KOREA – CORÉE
Kyobo Book Centre Co. Ltd.
P.O. Box 1658, Kwang Hwa Moon
Seoul   Tel. 730.78.91
Telefax: 735.00.30

MALAYSIA – MALAISIE
Co-operative Bookshop Ltd.
University of Malaya
P.O. Box 1127, Jalan Pantai Baru
59700 Kuala Lumpur
Malaysia   Tel. 756.5000/756.5425
Telefax: 757.3661

NETHERLANDS – PAYS-BAS
SDU Uitgeverij
Christoffel Plantijnstraat 2
Postbus 20014
2500 EA's-Gravenhage   Tel. (070 3) 78.99.11
Voor bestellingen: Tel. (070 3) 78.98.80
Telefax: (070 3) 47.63.51

NEW ZEALAND
NOUVELLE-ZÉLANDE
Legislation Services
P.O. Box 12418
Thorndon, Wellington   Tel. (04) 496.5652
Telefax: (04) 496.5698

NORWAY – NORVÈGE
Narvesen Info Center – NIC
Bertrand Narvesens vei 2
P.O. Box 6125 Etterstad
0602 Oslo 6   Tel. (02) 57.33.00
Telefax: (02) 68.19.01

PAKISTAN
Mirza Book Agency
65 Shahrah Quaid-E-Azam
Lahore 3   Tel. 66.839
Telex: 44886 UBL PK. Attn: MIRZA BK

PORTUGAL
Livraria Portugal
Rua do Carmo 70-74
Apart. 2681
1117 Lisboa Codex   Tel.: (01) 347.49.82/3/4/5
Telefax: (01) 347.02.64

OECD PUBLICATIONS, 2 rue André-Pascal, 75775 PARIS CEDEX 16
PRINTED IN FRANCE
(81 92 02 1) ISBN 92-64-13791-2 - No. 46039 1992